DIAGNOSIS AND IMAGING OF CHRONIC PANCREATITIS

DIAGNOSIS AND IMAGING OF CHRONIC PANCREATITIS

KENNETH COENEGRACHTS,
HANS RIGAUTS,
VINCENT DE WILDE
AND
VINCENT DENOLIN

Nova Biomedical Books
New York

Copyright © 2009 by Nova Science Publishers, Inc.

All rights reserved. No part of this book may be reproduced, stored in a retrieval system or transmitted in any form or by any means: electronic, electrostatic, magnetic, tape, mechanical photocopying, recording or otherwise without the written permission of the Publisher.
For permission to use material from this book please contact us:
Telephone 631-231-7269; Fax 631-231-8175
Web Site: http://www.novapublishers.com

NOTICE TO THE READER

The Publisher has taken reasonable care in the preparation of this book, but makes no expressed or implied warranty of any kind and assumes no responsibility for any errors or omissions. No liability is assumed for incidental or consequential damages in connection with or arising out of information contained in this book. The Publisher shall not be liable for any special, consequential, or exemplary damages resulting, in whole or in part, from the readers' use of, or reliance upon, this material.

Independent verification should be sought for any data, advice or recommendations contained in this book. In addition, no responsibility is assumed by the publisher for any injury and/or damage to persons or property arising from any methods, products, instructions, ideas or otherwise contained in this publication.

This publication is designed to provide accurate and authoritative information with regard to the subject matter covered herein. It is sold with the clear understanding that the Publisher is not engaged in rendering legal or any other professional services. If legal or any other expert assistance is required, the services of a competent person should be sought. FROM A DECLARATION OF PARTICIPANTS JOINTLY ADOPTED BY A COMMITTEE OF THE AMERICAN BAR ASSOCIATION AND A COMMITTEE OF PUBLISHERS.

Library of Congress Cataloging-in-Publication Data

Diagnosis and imaging of chronic pancreatitis / Kenneth Coenegrachts ... [et al.] (authors).
  p. ; cm.
Includes bibliographical references and index.
ISBN 978-1-60456-691-8 (softcover)
1. Pancreatitis--Imaging. 2. Pancreatitis--Diagnosis. 3. Pancreas--Cancer--Diagnosis. I. Coenegrachts, Kenneth.
[DNLM: 1. Pancreatitis--diagnosis. 2. Chronic Disease. 3. Diagnosis, Differential. 4. Diagnostic Imaging. 5. Pancreatic Neoplasms--diagnosis. WI 805 D5355 2008]
RC858.P35D53 2008
616.99'437075--dc22
                                     2008015194

Published by Nova Science Publishers, Inc. ✢ *New York*

Contents

Preface

Chapter I   Early Chronic Pancreatitis

Chapter II   Pancreatic Cancer

Chapter III   Differentiation of an Early Neoplastic and Inflammatory Mass in Chronic Pancreatitis

Chapter IV   Dorsal Extension of Resectable Pancreatic Cancer

Chapter V   Future Developments in the Diagnosis of Pancreatic Disease

Conclusion

References

Index

Preface

The insidious nature of disease taken into account, the majority of patients with chronic or malignant pancreatic disease present late in their course and even with early diagnosis, mortality rates of pancreatic cancer are high.
In anticipation of a better understanding of the molecular biology and the epigenesis in the origin and progression of disease, benign and malignant as well, the most challenging items in the diagnosis and management reside at present in endoscopic and radiological pancreatic imaging.
In these the diagnosis of early chronic pancreatitis, of early pancreatic cancer, the differentiation of a pancreatic mass in the setting of chronic pancreatitis and the accurate staging of potentially resectable pancreatic cancer with respect to the dorsal extension are of utmost importance. Focus in this chapter is on the diagnostic and imaging challenges of chronic pancreatitis and the differentiation with pancreatic cancer in an early stage.

Chapter I

Early Chronic Pancreatitis

Chronic pancreatitis (CP) is a disease of prolonged inflammation, induced by the fibrogenic pancreatic stellate cells and turning into irreversible morphologic and/or functional disturbances [1, 2, 3]. The triggers, thresholds, immunologic response and mechanisms of CP remain unclear and are still under investigation.[4] Despite marked progress in diagnostic tools and imaging methods there is no consensus in the grading of CP up till now. The various classification systems include the Marseilles (1963), Cambridge (1984), Marseilles (1984), Rome (1988), Chari (1994), Ammann (1997) and ABC system (2002).[5, 6, 7, 8, 9, 10, 11]. The diagnosis of CP at an early stage remains the biggest clinical challenge. Tissue biopsy, considered to be the gold standard [12, 13, 14], is generally not performed in view of the high complication rate [14] and may not be diagnostic in case of a patchy distribution of the histological lesions.[15] On the other hand currently available imaging modalities (Endoscopic Retrograde Pancreatography (ERP), Computed Tomography (CT), Endoscopic UltraSound (EUS), Magnetic Resonance Imaging (MRI)) have limited sensitivity and/or specificity for early CP and rely on quantitative criteria. As a consequence efforts are being made to search for biological and functional markers of early-stage CP [16, 17].

ERP has long been considered the gold standard imaging procedure for CP but gives no information with regard to parenchymal abnormalities [18, 19, 20].

The value of CT in identifying early ductal and parenchymal changes is negligible.[18, 21, 22, 23]. Endoscopic ultrasound is superior to the other imaging techniques with CP being likely once 5 of more criteria out of 9 to 11 have been reached.[24] The EUS criteria for CP are the presence of hyperechoic foci, hyperechoic strands, a lobular outer gland margin, lobularity, stones, calcifications, ductal dilation, side branch dilation, duct irregularity, hyperechoic duct margins, cysts, atrophy and a non-homogeneous echo pattern.[24] Not all criteria may be equally important and age-related changes as well may affect the diagnostic threshold.[25] In this respect the presence of intraductal calcifications on their own are highly suggestive of CP even in the absence of additional criteria and the widening of the pancreatic duct together with a hyperechogenic wall may be normal above the age of 70. As more criteria are reached, the specificity (positive predictive value) rises and the sensitivity (negative predictive value) lowers [24]. MRI of the pancreas in general uses a combination of T2-weighted (T2w) and T1-weighted (T1w) sequences. In most cases an MRI examination is started with T2w imaging in the axial plane. Additional coronal T2w imaging can be useful to depict the pancreatic and bile ducts more accurately. A T2w Half-Fourier Acquisition Single-Shot Turbo Spin Echo (HASTE) or Single-Shot-Fast Spin Echo (SS-FSE) sequence is a single-shot technique that acquires just over half of k-space in a single echo train, using k-space symmetry to reconstruct the image. The main advantage of the HASTE-sequence is its insensitivity to motion artifacts, even without breath-holding. The drawbacks of the HASTE-sequence include poorer Signal-to-Noise Ratio (SNR) when compared with multi-shot FSE-techniques, and blurring as a result of T2-decay during the long echo train. The resultant decreased sensitivity for detecting small, low-contrast lesions in the liver can be partially remedied by adding fat-suppression. These drawbacks, however, are not considered diagnostically significant when combined with the information obtained from the T1w unenhanced and dynamic contrast-enhanced sequences [26]. Nonetheless, non-fat-suppressed T2w imaging allows an improved evaluation of the fat stranding when compared with fat-suppressed imaging. For very ill patients who are unable to tolerate breath-holding, breathing-independent sequences using single-shot techniques such as T2w HASTE or SS-FSE are very useful.

In most cases T2w imaging is combined with so-called MRCP images. MRCP imaging uses heavily T2w imaging displaying only fluid. This allows depiction of the bile ducts and pancreatic ducts. Dynamic MRCP imaging furthermore allows evaluation of the repetitive contractions at the level of the sphincter of Oddi.

Concerning T1w imaging, two types of breath-hold sequences are mostly employed [26]:

1   In-and-out-of-phase gradient-echo (GE) imaging

2   Three-dimensional T1w GE imaging with fat-suppression

Fat-Suppression (FS) results in improvement in the (contrast-enhanced) dynamic range of non-fatty tissues, enhancing the contrast between different tissues and reducing motion artifacts from high signal intensity fat. The in-phase GE-sequence and T1w FS GE sequence are excellent for demonstrating areas of low signal intensity indicating pathologic changes within a normal spontaneously hyperintense pancreatic parenchyma. The decreased signal intensity on T1w FS images reflects the loss of soluble proteins in the acini of the pancreas. To our experience this finding is often more helpful when compared with the information obtained with contrast-enhanced T1w imaging.

Magnetic Resonance Imaging in the Diagnosis of Chronic Pancreatitis

The diagnosis of CP on MRI is based on signal intensity and enhancement changes as well as on morphologic abnormalities in the pancreatic parenchyma, pancreatic duct, and biliary tract. The imaging features of CP can be divided into early and late findings. Early findings include low-signal-intensity pancreas on T1w FS images, decreased and delayed enhancement after IV contrast administration, and dilated side branches. Late findings include parenchymal atrophy or enlargement, pseudocysts, and dilatation and beading of the pancreatic duct often with intraductal calcifications.

MRI allows early recognition of CP based on changes in pancreatic signal intensity; these changes are best visualized on unenhanced and gadolinium-enhanced T1w FS images. Chronic inflammation and fibrosis diminish the proteinaceous fluid content of the pancreas, resulting in the loss of the usual high signal intensity on T1w FS images. The normal pancreas enhances uniformly and intensely on late arterial phase contrast-enhanced T1w FS images and exhibits rapid washout of gadolinium on subsequent images. In contrast, a pancreas with chronic fibrosis and glandular atrophy exhibits decreased and heterogeneous enhancement on late arterial phase images and increased relative enhancement on delayed images [27].

Until recently, the role of MRCP in cases of CP was limited to diagnosis and follow-up of advanced cases.[28, 29] Owing to spatial resolution that is lower than that of ERP, ductal abnormalities in cases of mild CP cannot be assessed at

MRCP. Side branches usually are depicted only when dilated. Moreover, the condition in which the pancreatic ductal system is demonstrated at MRCP differs from that in which it is depicted during ERP. Indeed, in ERP, retrograde injection of contrast medium creates enlargement of the ducts, whereas in MRCP, the physiologic or physiopathologic ductal liquid content is demonstrated.

ERP by many is the standard of reference for imaging the pancreaticobiliary system because of its high image resolution and the advantage of allowing therapeutic intervention. ERP is useful especially for depicting side branch changes of early CP. Today, diagnostic ERP is challenged by MRCP, which is a noninvasive diagnostic alternative to ERP for the morphologic evaluation of normal and diseased pancreatic ducts.[28, 29, 30, 31] The administration of secretin during MRCP may help detect subtle side branch abnormalities and allows noninvasive assessment of exocrine pancreatic function. Duct abnormalities such as dilatation, irregularity, and stones and complications of CP such as pseudocysts are best depicted by thin-section T2w and thick-slab T2w MRCP images. MRCP is accurate in depicting strictures of the pancreatic duct or biliary tract. The beaded main pancreatic duct with its dilated side branches may have a chain-of-lakes appearance when more extensive.

CT is more sensitive than MRI for the detection of calcifications associated with CP; however, MRI best depicts intraductal stones and duct obstruction. Unlike ERP, MRCP can show the dilated duct upstream from an obstructing stone. Nevertheless, visualizing intraductal stones not surrounded by fluid may be difficult on MRI [32].

Recent technical issues with regard to MRCP include monitoring of pancreatic flow dynamics and duodenal filling after pancreatic hormonal stimulation with secretin. This is made possible by the advent of single-shot heavily T2w MRI sequences. This technique improves depiction of the pancreatic ducts and may allow estimation of pancreatic exocrine reserve [33]. Cappeliez O. et al. [34] compared duodenal filling as measured on MRCP obtained 10 minutes after secretin injection with biochemical parameters in pure pancreatic juice (PPJ) collected during the intraductal secretin test.

Dynamic variations in main pancreatic ductal diameter after secretin stimulation can be monitored. Measurable dilatation of the main pancreatic duct is mostly observed within 2–6 minutes of secretin injection. [34] This is explained by a secretin-stimulated increase in fluid secretion by the ductal cells in the ductal system and by simultaneously increased tonus of the sphincter of Oddi during the first 5 minutes, which inhibits the release of fluid through the papilla of Vater. [35] After that time, the tonus of the sphincter decreases, and the caliber of the main pancreatic duct returns to the baseline value as the pancreatic juice flows out through the papilla and progressively fills the duodenum. All main pancreatic ductal diameters measured on the dynamic MRI studies were significantly higher in patients with CP in the study by Cappeliez et al. [34]. Furthermore, the time to reach peak ductal diameter was longer, and the percentage increase in diameter was lower in patients with CP than in control patients. This probably reflects the fibrotic process involving pancreatic parenchyma in patients with CP. Cappeliez et al. [34] provide additional data regarding the relevance of duodenal filling observed during MRCP after secretin stimulation. Until now, there has been only speculation that duodenal filling could be correlated with exocrine pancreatic function [33]. Currently, the most valuable pancreatic function tests are the duodenal and intraductal secretin tests with sampling of duodenal juice or PPJ. [36, 37, 38, 39] With these invasive techniques, the best evaluation of the pancreatic exocrine function is given by measuring bicarbonate output and concentration in PPJ collected after secretin stimulation [37, 40, 41].

Cappeliez O. et al. [34] indicate a strong association between reduced duodenal filling and impaired pancreatic exocrine function. Patients with reduced duodenal filling observed at MRCP are 17.6 times more likely to have deficient pancreatic function (ie, ≤50% of normal function) than are patients with normal duodenal filling. By considering duodenal filling alone in patients with reduced pancreatic function, reduced duodenal filling is specific (87%) but less sensitive (72%) for detection of impaired pancreatic exocrine function; therefore, normal duodenal filling seen at MRCP after secretin stimulation does not exclude reduced pancreatic exocrine function.

Although some investigators [42, 43, 44] have shown a correlation between secretin stimulation test and ERP results in patients with CP, others [34, 45] have shown that exocrine pancreatic function as assessed with PPJ analysis (and with findings of duodenal filling, in our study) may be normal in patients with abnormal ERP findings and vice versa, with discordant results in 12%–29% of cases [43, 44, 45].

Matos C. et al. [46] describe progressive hydrographic enhancement of the pancreatic parenchyma, termed acinar filling, during dynamic secretin MRCP studies probably being a specific, although insensitive, finding of early CP. The cause of this acinar filling remains unclear, with subtle or no ductal changes on ERCP and without calcifications. However, Matos C. et al. [46] state that acinar filling might illustrate the ductal and tissue hypertension that have been described in humans [47] and in animal models in the early stages of CP.[48, 49] Ductal and tissue hypertension are due to both outflow impairment and a lack of compliance of the diseased pancreas. Progressive acinar filling could represent fluid leakage caused by increased ductal and tissue pressure in a pancreas that has lost its elasticity [47, 50].

Perfusion-Based Contrast-Enhanced MRI of the Pancreas

In a prospective study by K.Coenegrachts et al. [51], the potential of a non-invasive technique, namely perfusion-based contrast-enhanced MRI, has been explored as a diagnostic tool for CP (Figure 1). The rationale for this study came from the observation of a decreased pancreatic tissue perfusion in animal studies [52, 53], as well as in humans with CP.[54, 55] This study was performed on a 1.5T MRI scanner (Intera, Philips, Best, The Netherlands), using the synergy body phased-array coil. The imaging protocol consisted of a scout acquisition, a reference scan for the use of Sensitivity Encoding (SENSE) reconstruction in subsequent acquisitions and coronal T2-weighted Half-Fourier Turbo Spin Echo (Haste) acquisitions. The Haste images were used to accurately localize the pancreatic parenchyma in all subjects and to position the 3D imaging volume on the pancreas. The perfusion study was performed with a series of 3D RF spoiled T1w gradient echo acquisitions.

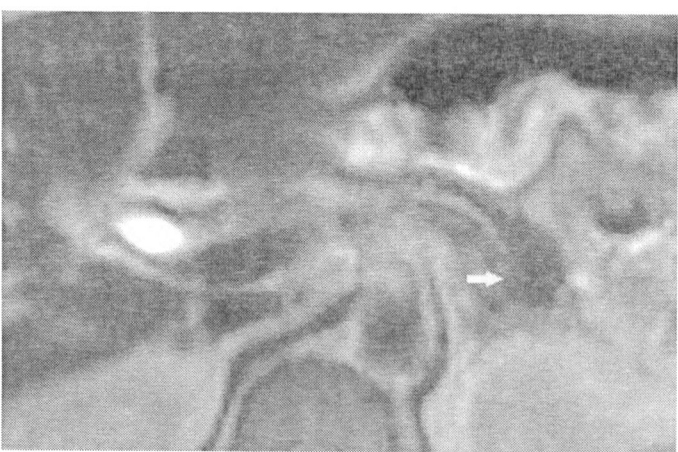

Figure 1a. T2w TSE (short TE) MRI-sequence displaying an area of pathologic signal intensity changes (white arrow) between normal and pathologic (proximal part of pancreatic tail) pancreatic parenchyma.

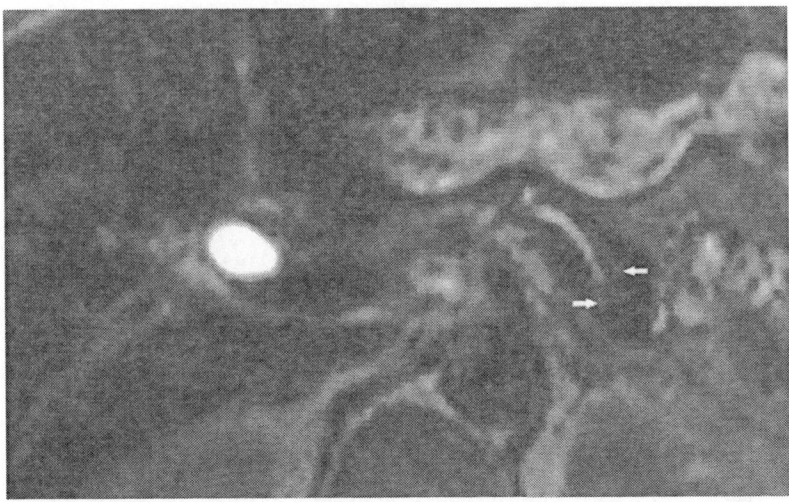

Figure 1b. T2w TSE (long TE) MRI-sequence displaying the above mentioned area of pathologic signal intensity changes. In this area some dilated side branches (white arrows) can be detected.

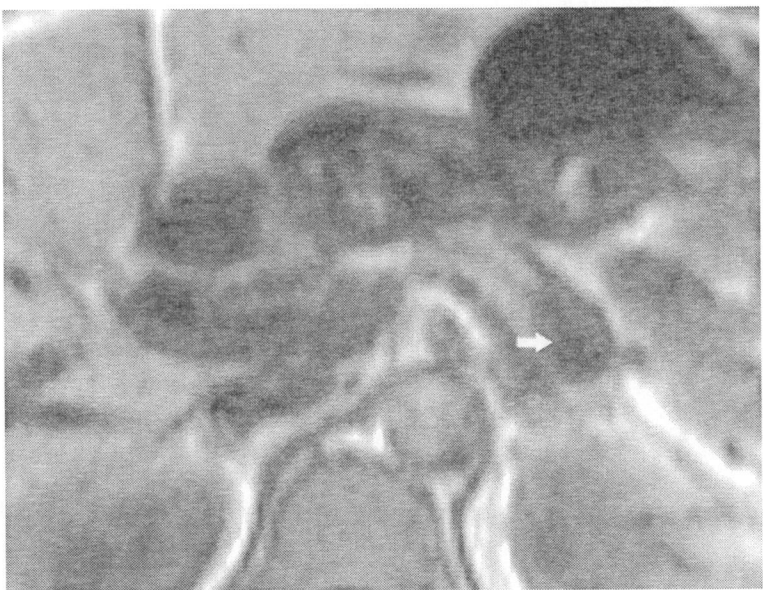

Figure 1c. T1w GE MRI-sequence before IV injection of contrast agent and without fat suppression also displays the above mentioned area of pathologic signal intensity changes (white arrow).

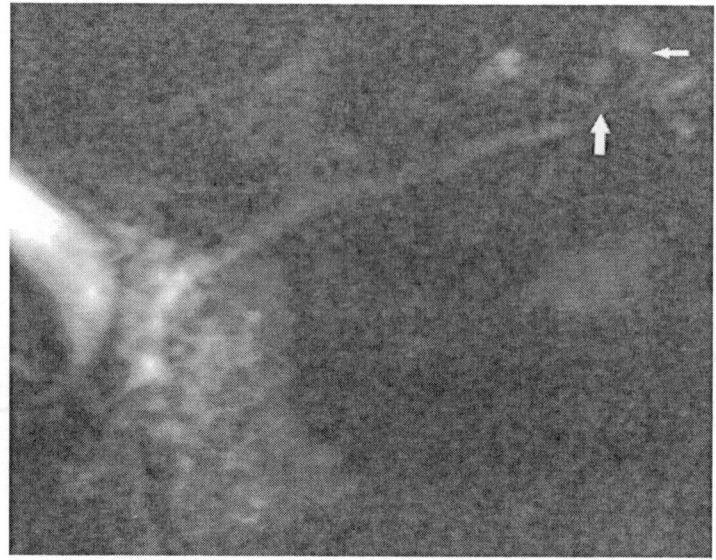

Figure 1d. MRCP-sequence displays a focal distinctive narrowing of the main pancreatic duct and accompanying dilated side branches (white arrows) at the level of the above mentioned signal intensity changes.

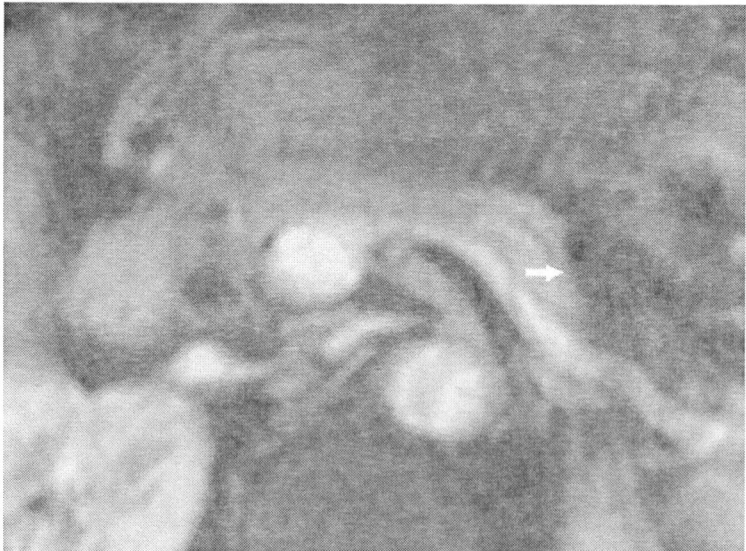

Figure 1e.

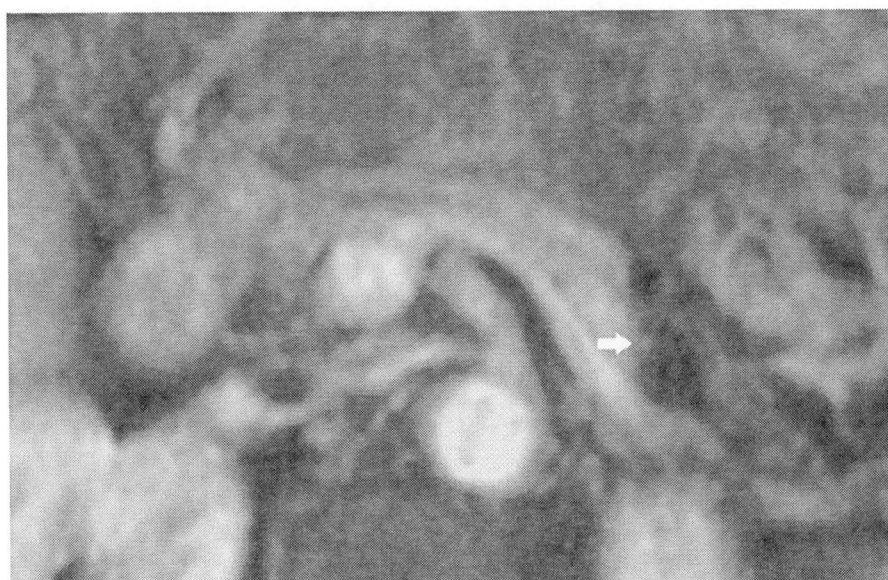

Figure 1f.

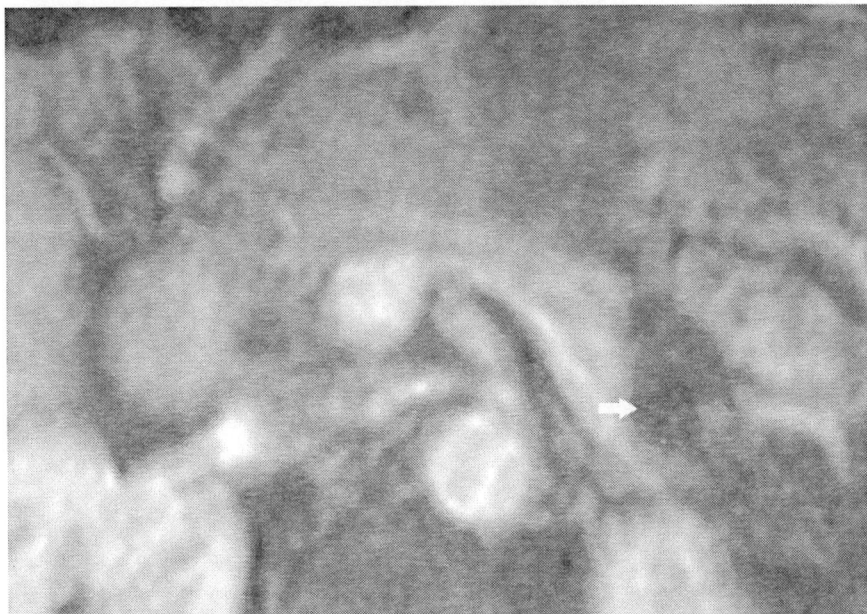

Figure 1g.

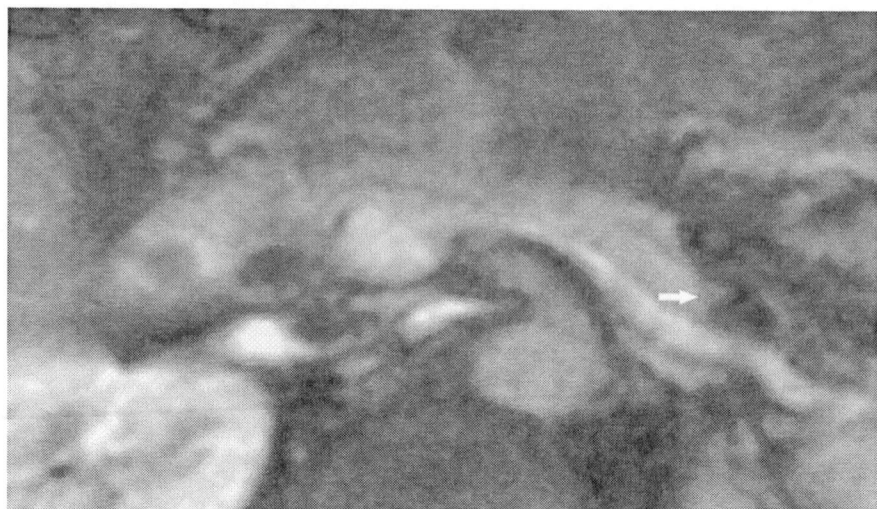

Figure 1h.

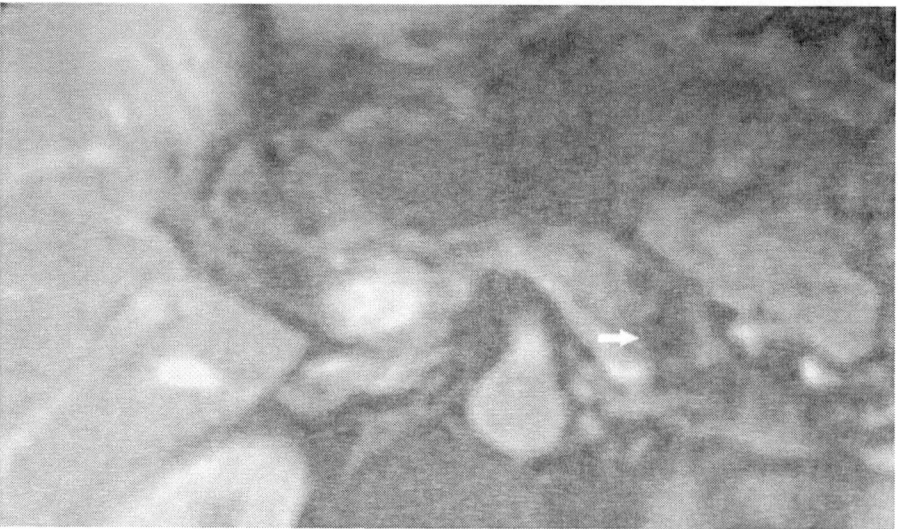

Figure 1i.

Figure 1e-i. T1w GE MRI-sequence with fat suppression during IV injection of contrast agent. Dynamic "perfusion-based" MRI was performed obtaining images of the entire pancreatic parenchyma every 2 seconds (modified sequence from the one used in earlier study by Coenegrachts K. et al. reference [51]) displaying a gradually increasing contrast-enhancement at the level of the above mentioned signal intensity changes. Further study needs to be done to find a reliable threshold (reliable Time-Intensity-Curve) for the differentiation between focal chronic pancreatitis and a focal pancreatic cancer.

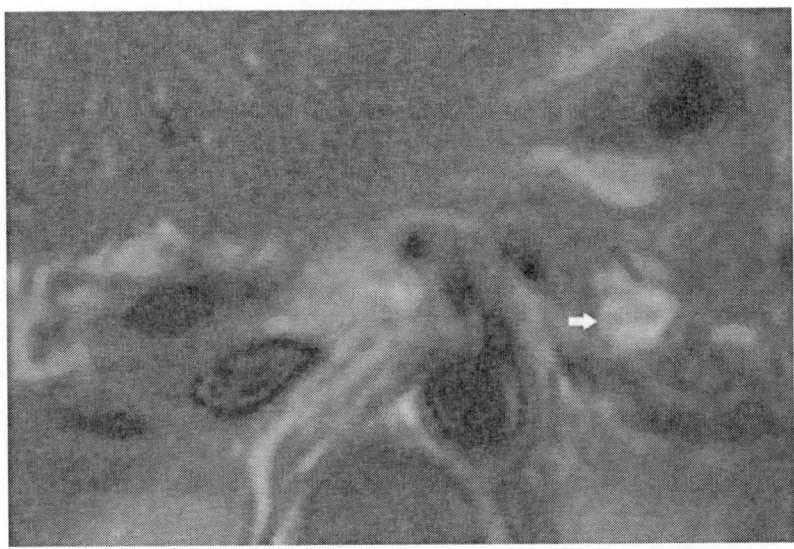

Figure 1j. Follow-up T2w TSE (short TE) MRI-sequence after two weeks displaying a strong hyperintense signal (white arrow) at the earlier detected level of pathologic signal intensity change. This finding suggests evolution toward development of a pseudocyst.

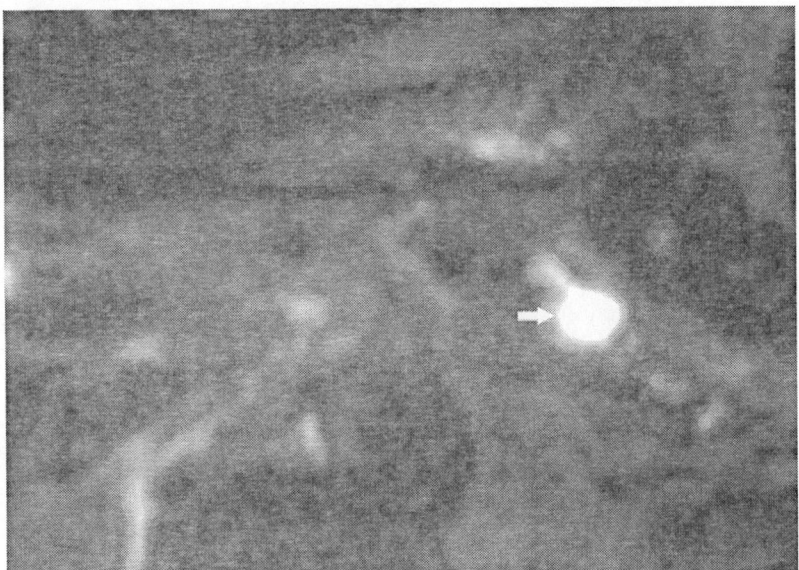

Figure 1k. Follow-up T2w TSE (long TE) MRI-sequence after two weeks again displaying a strong hyperintense signal compatible with fluid (pseudocyst).

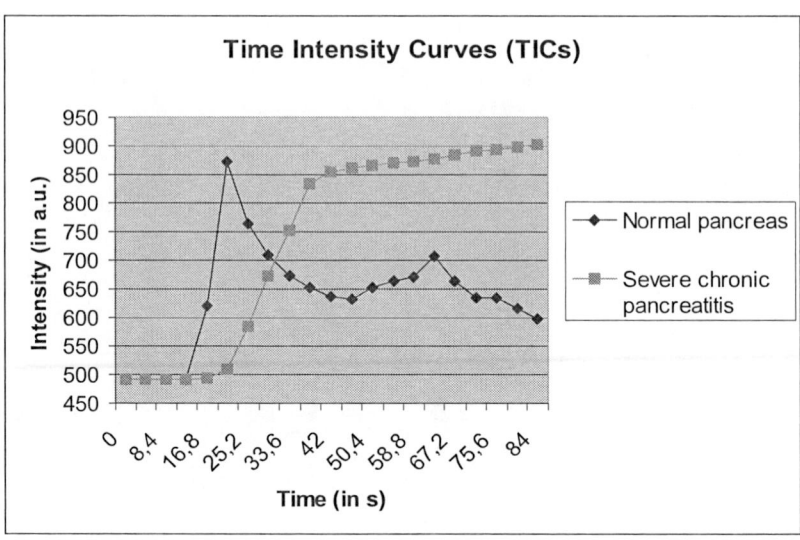

Figure 2. shows a typical Time Intensity Curve (TIC) in a healthy subject and in a patient with severe chronic pancreatitis. The first and second pass of contrast material can clearly be appreciated in the healthy subject.

A dose of 0.1mmol/kg Gd-DTPA (Omniscan®, Nycomed, Ireland) contrast agent was used followed by a bolus of 20 ml of physiologic saline (NaCl 0,9%). The patient inclusion criteria for moderate to severe CP were imaging findings considered diagnostic of moderate to severe CP (Cambridge classification type II or III) with or without a concommittant functional exocrine or endocrine insufficiency. Criteria for exocrine insufficiency were an abnormal mixed triglycerides breathing test and/or the presence of abnormal fecal fat measurements. Criteria for endocrine insufficiency were an abnormal oral glucose tolerance test. Patients with prior abdominal surgery were excluded.

Patients with thrombosis or obstruction in the portal vein and its branches were excluded from the study. The signal enhancement curve from data in the aorta was used to check for unknown cardiovascular pathologies with influence on the aortic flow. In all cases the complete first pass of the bolus was visualized. Three Regions-Of-Interest (ROIs) (at the level of pancreatic head, body and tail respectively) could be chosen in all subjects. In patients suffering from CP, some dilated side branches were inevitably included within the ROI. Regions of interest (ROIs) were selected in the pancreatic head, body and tail and enhancement curves (Time-Intensity-Curves (TICs)) were calculated. Typical TICs in the pancreas of both a volunteer and a patient with CP are shown in figure 2. In the volunteer, the enhancement curve shows the baseline signal prior to the arrival of the contrast agent in the pancreatic parenchyma and an earlier and steeper increase in signal intensity during the early phase of contrast bolus when compared with the patient suffering from CP. Semi-quantitative parameters were calculated from the TICs in the pancreas of both healthy volunteers and patients with moderate to severe CP. The purpose was to compare the perfusion-related data in both groups. This is considered a first step towards a possible protocol for perfusion-based contrast-enhanced MRI for the diagnosis of early CP.

A first reason to use the 3D T1w FS GE technique is the better spatial resolution when compared, e.g. to T2*w perfusion acquisitions. In addition, bowel loops within the imaging volume don not induce susceptibility artefacts. The 3D volume included the complete pancreatic parenchyma and different parts of the pancreas were readily distinguished. A good spatial resolution is crucial for adequate placement of the different ROIs at the level of the pancreatic parenchyma. Especially in patients with moderate to severe CP, there can be a pronounced atrophy of the pancreatic parenchyma. A good spatial resolution is therefore a determining factor for the practical applicability of the technique. The dynamic 3D acquisition allows a temporal resolution of 4.2 sec per 3D-stack. It remains to be studied whether a shorter acquisition time, when using as an example a 2D gradient echo measurement, would change the values of the perfusion parameters.

Two parameters were found promising in this regard: the Time-to-Inflow Deceleration (TID) and the wash-in rate (Figure 3). The TID in the pancreatic head, body and tail of patients with CP is significantly longer than in volunteers. The wash-in rate at the level of the pancreatic head and body is significantly slower in patients with CP. These findings might be explained by a combination of microcirculatory disturbances, changes in compliance/elasticity of the pancreatic parenchyma, by an increased tissue pancreatic interstitial pressure and possibly also by an important diffusion of the contrast agent into the pancreatic parenchyma. A laser Doppler flow study, performed in patients with alcoholic pancreatitis undergoing laparatomy for pancreatic head resection, showed a significantly decreased pancreatic blood flow and also alterations in the blood flow wave or pulsatile index as compared to normal controls [55].

In a series of studies performed in both animals with experimentally induced CP as well as in patients with CP, Reber and coworkers demonstrated a decreased pancreatic perfusion but also an increased pancreatic interstitial pressure as compared to controls.[52] According to the latter authors, stimulation of the pancreas by the administration of secretin and cholecystokinin leads to an increase in blood flow in the normal pancreas but to a further reduction in blood flow and a further increase in interstitial pressure when dealing with CP. Duct decompression, especially by surgical pancreaticojejunostomy, improves pancreatic blood flow, decreases interstitial pressure, and prevents any further deterioration on pancreatic secretagogue stimulation [56].

When using the non-specific contrast agents, the enhancement slope always expresses tissue vascularisation given by the number and dimension of vessels and capillary permeability.[57, 58] During the first pass, approximately 50% of the contrast agent (or even more in pathologic tissues) enters the interstitial space through the capillary network. The complete enhancement curve (TIC) is therefore mainly determined by the capillary permeability and the composition of the interstitial space. [59] The use of blood pool agents, i.e. contrast agents that remain for a much longer time in the vessels, visualises the perfusion more selectively [60].

Differences in signal intensity on fat-suppressed, T1-weighted images and percent contrast enhancement on dynamic images have been previously observed between healthy persons and patients with CP.[27, 61, 62] Only in one recent study, two quantitative signs were described to characterize patients with an apparent "early or mild" CP by dynamic contrast-enhanced MRI.[63]

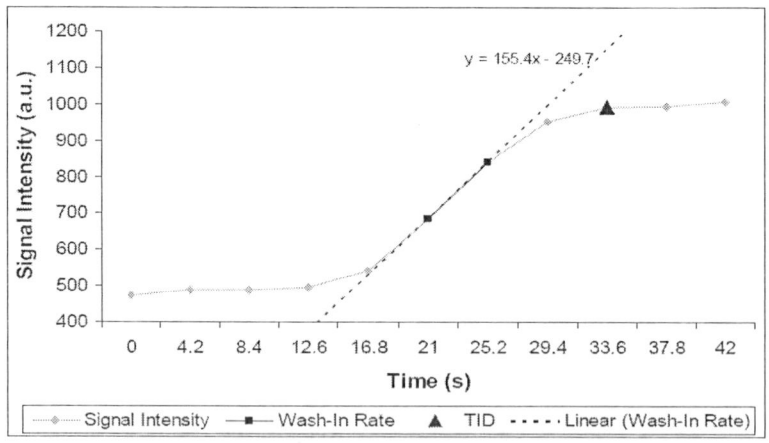

Figure 3. A TIC of a patient with chronic pancreatitis is shown, displaying how the Time-to-Inflow Deceleration (TID) parameter and wash-in are measured. The wash-in rate was defined as the maximal signal intensity gradient or slope that can be calculated between successive measured time points; the TID is the duration from the onset of the signal enhancement to the point where the wash-in rate decreases to less than 10% of its maximal value.

In this retrospective study, 24 patients with suspected early or mild CP, classified by imaging criteria of equivocal CP (ultrasound, computed tomography (CT) or ERCP) grading, had dynamic MRI that included unenhanced, arterial, early venous, and late venous phases of contrast enhancement. Twenty patients without pancreatic diseases also had the dynamic sequence as a control group. The signal intensity was measured at the pancreatic head, body, and tail on all phases, and for each, the signal intensity ratio (SIR, the signal intensity in postcontrast divided by that in precontrast) was calculated. Two radiologists independently reviewed the images of the patients with suspected early or mild CP for pancreatic morphologic abnormalities without knowing the results of signal intensity measurements. Patients with CP had a relative signal enhancement of 1.65 ± 0.23 in the arterial phase. This was significantly lower than the corresponding value in normal controls, 1.89 ± 0.31, and that was also significantly lower than in the early venous phase: 1.75 ± 0.22. The presence of a signal intensity ratio < 1.73 in the arterial phase and/or a delayed peak enhancement after contrast had a sensitivity of 92% and a specificity of 75% for early CP. This is significantly higher than the 50% sensitivity for diagnosis based on morphological abnormalities alone.[64] The parameters were calculated from 3 successive 3D GE acquisitions (lasting 20s each) during the injection of a contrast agent. In this study we found two quantitative signs of suspected early or mild CP on dynamic contrast-enhanced MRI. The arterial phase SIR of the pancreatitis group was significantly lower than that of the control group ($P < 0.01$). Additionally, enhancement in the pancreatitis group was greatest in the early or late venous phase, rather than in the arterial phase, as in the control group ($P < 0.05$). The sensitivity of 92% for diagnosing suspected early or mild CP by measuring pancreatic signal intensity on dynamic contrast-enhanced images was significantly higher than the sensitivity of 50% depending on visible pancreatic morphologic changes ($P < 0.05$). Additionally, we found that pancreatic morphologic abnormalities did not correlate significantly with pancreatic enhancement measurements. This indicates that abnormal pancreatic enhancement may precede or be independent of pancreatic morphologic abnormalities. Our population with suspected early or mild CP had unenhanced pancreatic signal intensity that was not significantly different from that of our control group. Measuring pancreatic signal intensity on gadolinium chelate dynamic MRI is helpful for diagnosing early or mild CP, especially before apparent pancreatic morphologic or signal intensity changes are present. This method is different from present approach. Therefore the results cannot be correlated with the values obtained in this work. In addition, also the selection of patients was different.

Endoscopic Ultrasound

EUS has developed significantly over the last two decades and has had a considerable impact on the imaging and staging of mass lesions within or in close proximity to the gastrointestinal (GI) tract. In conjunction with conventional imaging such as helical CT and MRI, among others some indications for EUS include assessing suspected pancreatic lesions that are either equivocal or not seen on conventional imaging and staging malignant tumors of the pancreas prior to surgery or oncological treatment. The introduction of linear scanning instruments has also allowed tissue sampling of suspicious lesions under real time EUS control to become feasible (EUS-guided fine needle aspiration or FNA), and in many cases can be performed more safely than with conventional techniques [65].

Endoscopic Ultrasound in the Diagnosis of Chronic Pancreatitis

EUS has been proposed as a diagnostic test for early CP. A number of features of CP that might not be obvious on other imaging or functional tests can be demonstrated on EUS, including hyperechoic foci, hyperechoic strands, lobularity, cysts, calcification, stones, ductal dilatation, side branch dilatation, ductal irregularity, and hyperechoic duct margins.[24] Currently, it is generally accepted that the presence of five or more of the above criteria make the diagnosis of CP likely, but the significance of one to four criteria remains unclear and there is a need for a reliable gold standard for diagnosing CP. Studies comparing EUS criteria for CP with EUS-guided FNA cytology are ongoing. Two other factors must be taken into account when diagnosing CP based on EUS criteria. All criteria may not be equally important. For example, the presence of intraductal calcifications alone is highly suggestive of CP even in the absence of other criteria. In addition, there are age-related changes in the pancreas that may affect the diagnostic threshold.[25] The pancreatic duct becomes progressively wider with hyperechogenic wall as the individual ages. A 4 mm main pancreatic duct may be normal for a 70-year-old, but abnormal for a 30-year-old. Currently, there is no accepted scoring system that factors in these effects. One common practice is to require a higher threshold (e.g., 5 or more criteria for older individuals) and a lower threshold (e.g. 4 or more criteria for a younger individual). EUS criteria other than being solely quantified should also be correlated to the patient's clinical history along with the presence of risk factors (ethanol, smoking) [24].

Endoscopic Ultrasound in the Diagnosis of Early Chronic Pancreatitis

The diagnosis of CP is based on clinical features, morphologic changes and functional abnormalities. In the early stages of the disease, the diagnosis remains challenging and agreement between various methods is poor. [18, 19, 66, 67] Functional tests probably miss the diagnosis in the early stages because of exocrine pancreas functional reserve. Imaging studies, such as CT, have poor resolution, especially in the initial stages. ERP is still considered the most accurate method of assessing ductal anatomy [13, 18]. However, parenchymal abnormalities can be missed and post-procedure acute pancreatitis may occur in 5-10% of patients.[68, 69] Although these exams may be good indicators in the advanced stages, the same is not true in early-stage disease. Therefore, a method able to assess the early stages of both parenchymal and ductal irregularities with minimal risk would be of great value. EUS generates high-resolution images of parenchymal and ductal structures without the use of contrast without risk of post-procedure pancreatitis and minimal risk of sedation. EUS can also be used to obtain pancreatic tissue and juice samples. [13, 18, 20, 67, 70, 71]

EUS provides better resolution images than US, CT and ERP. Hence, both parenchymal and ductal morphology can be assessed without fluoroscopy or contrast injection. It is therefore possible to assume that EUS might be able to detect abnormalities not previously seen by other methods. Its complication rate is similar to diagnostic upper gastrointestinal endoscopy [66, 72]. EUS criteria for pancreatic disease are useful but have some limitations. Abnormalities may be similar in acute and chronic disease and slight changes of CP may be seen in the elderly population secondary to fibrotic changes related to age.[20, 70] Pancreatic abnormalities depicted by EUS can possibly be asymptomatic; on the other hand, patients highly suspected of having CP might present only mild EUS pancreatitis.[73, 74, 75] Yusoff and Sahai [76] prospectively studied the effect of ethanol and other variables on the endosonographic appearance of the pancreas and found that the number of criteria correlated most strongly with ethanol ingestion and smoking history. Wiersema et al. [20] prospectively evaluated 69 patients and 20 controls to assess pancreatic EUS features, demonstrating that sensitivity and specificity were optimal when 3 or more criteria were found. For all forms of CP, sensitivity was 80% and specificity was 86%. When considering initial pancreatic disease, sensitivity was 86%. In the study by Sahai et al. [66] 126 patients underwent EUS followed by ERP. The prevalence of CP in the population studied was 76% with 47% having moderate to severe disease. The authors found that this diagnosis can be made with an 85% certainty when more than 2 criteria are present and moderate to severe forms when more than 6 features are seen. Moderate to severe CP is unlikely (negative predictive value greater than 85%) when less than 3 criteria are found. Independent features predictive of CP were the sum of the criteria and alcohol abuse. Catalano et al. [19] evaluated 80 patients with non-alcoholic, acute, recurrent pancreatitis by EUS, ERP and pancreatic juice examination. The agreement between EUS and, both the secretin test and ERP was excellent for normal and severe pancreatitis, but poor for mild to moderate disease. When at least 3 EUS features were used to diagnose CP, the sensitivity was 86% and specificity 98%. This prospective study compared EUS appearance in patients with and without alcohol abuse excluding those with suspicious or confirmed diagnosis of CP. When comparing alcoholic and non-alcoholic groups, they found that the mean number of criteria was significantly higher in the alcoholic group. This suggests that although asymptomatic, alcoholic patients might have pancreatic abnormalities, which may be missed by other procedures, and EUS might be useful in screening patients with suspected initial stage CP. Still related to such findings, we can also argue that EUS is able to show early structural damage to the pancreas. The threshold of features needed to diagnose CP can vary according to whether or not we wish to maximize sensitivity and specificity. Once EUS detects structural changes not detected by other diagnostic methods, follow-up is necessary in order to rule out whether or not these patients who have been diagnosed with mild CP by EUS will develop signs of pancreatic disease.[77] Patients presenting more than 1 and 2 EUS features of the Catalano and Sahai score systems, respectively, are at great risk of having CP [77].

There is now some evidence in the literature suggesting that these early changes detected by EUS correlate with the histological changes of CP and may predict progression to more advanced disease. The EUS diagnosis of CP relies on quantitative (more than qualitative) parenchymal and ductal criteria found during evaluation of the pancreas. It is generally accepted that, in the absence of any criteria, CP is unlikely, whereas in the presence of 5 or more criteria (out of 9-11)

CP is likely although ERP and pancreatic function tests may still be normal. The diagnostic significance of patients with fewer (1-4) criteria found on EUS is currently unclear, particularly when other diagnostic tests such as ERP and function testing are normal. In these cases, there is a potential for "over-diagnosis" of CP, since the EUS changes cannot be confirmed by other modalities.[24] One measure of early CP is whether a patient responds to pancreatic specific therapy. Walsh et al. [78] identified 43 patients who had characteristic symptoms of pancreatic disease but normal or equivocal US, CT or ERP. Those patients (16 patients), whose symptoms failed to respond to medical therapy (enzyme replacement, low fat diet, and at least 3 trials of bowel rest with total parenteral nutrition), underwent pancreatic resection. The histologic appearance in the pancreas of these patients showed subtle but distinct evidence of minimal-change CP. These changes were "focally" distributed throughout the gland and included lymphocytic cell infiltrates, intralobular and periductal fibrosis, and focal ductal dilation with inspissated protein plugs. Nine of the 16 patients had complete or significant improvement in pain after total pancreatectomy, whereas 5 did not respond and 1 died of unrelated causes. The histologic changes and response to pancreatectomy suggest that these patients had CP despite normal imaging and functional testing. However, a placebo response cannot be excluded. In the absence of a gold standard, diagnostic tests must meet other accepted criteria to be considered valuable. These include inter- and intra-observer reliability, correlation with other validated (albeit non-gold standard) tests of the disease, and prediction of response to therapy. EUS meets some, but not all of these criteria. A fundamental requirement for any test is reliability. When no gold standard is available, this is often measured as the degree to which practitioners agree on a diagnosis. Wiersema et al. [20] compared the degree of agreement among 3 experienced endosonographers reading individual criteria of CP. The agreement was 88% for hyperechoic foci, 94% for focal reduced echogenicity, 94% for lobularity, 83% for hyperechoic duct margins and 94% for duct irregularity. To further improve the reliability, an "International Working Group" has published a set of "Minimum Standard Terminology (MST)", including definitions, for many of the EUS criteria of CP.[79] Zimmerman et al. [80] and Dr. Brenda Hoffman (personal communication) reported the EUS criteria in comparison to the histologic features of CP in 34 patients who underwent EUS followed by pancreatectomy or open surgical biopsy (at the time of a lateral pancreatico-duodenostomy) (21 for CP, 13 for pancreatic adenocarcinoma). Overall, 68% of the patients met the histologic criteria for CP. The total number of EUS criteria present was predictive of histologic CP. The sensitivity and specificity were 87% and 64% using a threshold diagnosis for 3 or more criteria, 78% and 73% for 4 or more criteria, 60% and 83% for 5 or more criteria, and 43% and 91% for 6 or more criteria. From these results, it was concluded that a threshold of 4 or more criteria was the optimal threshold. Hollerbach et al. [81] reported their experience with EUS-FNA in CP. These authors evaluated 27 patients with CP and compared the results of EUS with 22-gauge needle FNA with the results of ERCP. EUS-FNA increased the negative predictive value to 100% and the specificity to 64%. EUS results were in agreement with regard to the severity of CP according to the Cambridge classification at ERP in 5 of 8 patients with grade I, 11 of 13 patients with grade II, and 10 of 10 patients with grade III disease. Complications in the form of mild acute pancreatitis occurred in 2 patients (7%). On the average, 2.3 needle passes were needed to obtain a sufficient amount of tissue for diagnosis. This study better supports the role of EUS-FNA "in ruling out" rather than " in ruling in" CP. However, it is already well known that a normal EUS examination virtually rules out CP in the appropriate clinical context. Larger needles, improvements in tissue processing, and molecular biology markers could, in the future, expand the application of EUS-FNA in patients with CP.

As with the comparison to ERP, it is unknown if EUS is more sensitive to mild changes of CP than functional testing or if it is overdiagnosing early CP.[24] The natural history may be the most definitive gold standard for early CP. A diagnosis of "mild" CP based on EUS, which then progresses to more severe CP as diagnosed by other tests (EUS positive, ERCP, positive functional test), is likely to be a correct diagnosis. Unfortunately, there are only limited data on the long-term natural history of "mild" CP diagnosed by EUS. Hastier et al. [82] reported the short-term (mean: 22 months) progression of pancreatic disease in 17 asymptomatic alcoholics with an abnormal EUS but a normal ERP. Follow-up EUS examinations for 12-38 months did not identify any progression to more overt (ERP positive) disease. It is likely, however, that patients who took more than 55 years (mean age of study patients was 55.5 years) to develop "mild" disease, require more than 2-3 years to progress from mild to more severe disease. A cross-sectional study of alcoholic patients with and without abdominal pain by Bhutani [74] showed that the EUS diagnosis of CP (4 or more criteria) was positive in 89% of alcoholics with abdominal pain but also in 58% of alcoholics without pain, and 0% of control patients (non-alcoholic, no abdominal pain). More recently, Kahl et al. [75] reported a subgroup of 38 patients with a history of chronic alcohol use and recurrent abdominal pain. At the time of enrollment in the study, 32 of 38 patients had an abnormal EUS but a normal ERP. After a median follow-up of 18 months (range: 6-25 months), 22 of 32 patients developed changes of CP at ERP (12 patients grade I and 10 patients grade II according to the Cambridge classification). Contrary to the study of Hastier et al. [82], Kahl et al. [77] observed ERP changes of CP in a short follow-up (18 months). The only significant differences between the 2 studies appeared to be the presence of alcoholic cirrhosis in Hastier's study and the presence of abdominal pain and recurrent pancreatitis in Kahl's study. Further long-term follow up data are needed.

Nonetheless, there are also several disadvantages of EUS. EUS still remains confined to very few centers, and it is not widely available. Parada et al. [83] retrospectively reviewed the indications for EUS at three major EUS centers. Based on these data, they calculated the hypothetical demand for EUS in the United States to be 79,572 per year for all indications. Second, the value of EUS is directly proportional to the training, skill, and experience of the endosonographer. Virtually all of the data and published information pertaining to EUS are the work of a relatively small group of experts. Third, the principal concern in using EUS for the diagnosis of CP is the possibility that it may overdiagnose the features of CP, causing patients to be falsely diagnosed with CP when they do not have pancreatic disease. Because experts cannot agree on a gold standard for the diagnosis of CP, it has been difficult to determine the extent to which overdiagnosis occurs. In patients with EUS evidence of changes of CP but a normal secretin test or a normal ERP, it is not clear whether the EUS is more sensitive for early changes or if it is truly overdiagnosing CP [84].

Chapter II

Pancreatic Cancer

Pancreatic cancer is the most deadly of all gastrointestinal malignancies, the fourth leading cause of cancer-related deaths in the United States and has a very poor prognosis; almost all pancreatic cancer patients will die from this disease. The 5-year survival rate is less than 5%.[85] Pancreatic cancer is a major health problem for several reasons: the aggressive behavior of the tumor and the relative frequency which appears to be increasing; approximately 30,000 new cases in 2002 and about 32,000 in 2004 were diagnosed in the United States.[85] As pancreatic mass lesions are aggressive neoplasms, patients would benefit from early detection, diagnosis, and surgical intervention [86, 87].

Unfortunately most patients present late in the course of their disease with advanced cancer either locally or with metastatic spread.[88, 89] Even though surgery represents the only chance for cure, at the time of diagnosis only 10 to 25% (in the more optimistic series) of pancreatic cancer patients will be eligible for potentially curative resection [89, 90, 91, 92] and the prognosis remains dismal even for patients with potentially curative resections. This is clearly demonstrated by a 5-year survival rate which does not surpass 20% even after surgical resection.[93, 94, 95] Furthermore, considering the high cost of major pancreatic surgery, not only in terms of money but also in terms of morbidity and mortality even in the most experienced surgical hands [96, 97], it is clear that all efforts must be oriented towards the need for an early diagnosis and towards reliably identifying patients who really can benefit from major surgical intervention. A recent study [98] indeed found that a complete resection with negative margins could be achieved in almost half of 53 patients with suspicion of locoregional pancreatic cancer when state-of-the-art preoperative imaging is used.

Chapter III

Differentiation of an Early Neoplastic and Inflammatory Mass in Chronic Pancreatitis

Patients with CP have an increased risk of pancreatic cancer, most probably due to increased cell turnover and defective DNA repair with loss of p16 expression and K-ras mutations [99, 100].

Allowing for the relationship between CP and pancreatic cancer to differentiate between a neoplastic and inflammatory pancreatic mass may be extremely difficult, even in view of the different clinical histories and features. A further confounding factor is that some pancreatic cancers are associated with a marked desmoplastic reaction in the pancreas, creating peritumour fibrosis [101].

Microscopically, desmoplastic change leads to hypovascularity of pancreatic ductal adenocarcinomas. Another reason for hypovascularity of ductal adenocarcinomas is vascular encasement, causing arterial stenosis or obstruction.[102] On the contrary, an inflammatory pancreatic mass which is a focal swelling of the pancreas, consists of inflammatory changes such as interlobular fibrosis and chronic inflammatory infiltrate around lobules and ducts.[103] Those inflammatory changes usually require blood flow and result in hypervascularity. Therefore most inflammatory masses show more vascularity than pancreatic adenocarcinomas. However, severe fibrosis can replace pancreatic acinar cells and inhibit vascular development in an inflammatory lesion which is probably the reason why a focal inflammatory pancreatic mass can be hypovascular [104].

Nonetheless, tissue diagnosis (cytologic or histologic examination) often is used in the differentiation of focal CP and pancreatic adenocarcinoma, with EUS-guided fine-needle aspiration (EUS-FNA) usually performed. EUS-FNA is becoming the standard for obtaining cytologic diagnosis, although the sensitivity of EUS-FNA for the differential diagnosis of a focal pancreatic mass is variable in the literature, being as low as 75% in some studies [105]. Moreover, the sensitivity was reported to be unacceptably lower (about 54%) in the context of focal CP, whereas surgical resection was still necessary to confirm the diagnosis [106].

Overall, imaging examinations (CT, MRI, PET, EUS) and EUS FNA have limited success in differentiating between focal CP and pancreatic adenocarcinoma [107].

General CT and MRI Features in the Diagnosis of Pancreatic Adenocarcinoma

Dilatation of the main pancreatic duct, parenchymal atrophy, pancreatic calcification, fluid collection, focal pancreatic enlargement (pancreatic mass due to CP), biliary ductal dilatation, and changes in attenuation in peripancreatic fat or fascia are frequent findings in patients with CP.[108] These findings are also often seen as secondary changes in patients with pancreatic adenocarcinoma.[109] These overlaps of imaging findings make it difficult to distinguish a focal pancreatic mass due to CP from a pancreatic adenocarcinoma or other tumors.

Helical CT and dynamic MRI have been reported useful for detecting and characterizing pancreatic cancers.[110, 111, 112, 113] Pancreatic duct adenocarcinoma is usually hypovascular and appears as a hypoenhanced lesion relative to surrounding pancreatic parenchyma on pancreatic phase images of helical CT and on dynamic MRI.[111, 112] However, these studies didn't focus on early pancreatic cancer. Johnson and Outwater [110] found that masses of pancreatic adenocarcinoma and those due to CP showed more gradual progressive enhancement on dynamic MRI than did normal pancreatic parenchyma, and they histologically found abundant fibrosis in both pathologic conditions, which was thought to account for the similar imaging appearances of the two kinds of masses. Especially when differentiating early focal CP and early pancreatic cancer, this causes differential diagnostic problems.

Computed Tomography in the Differentiation of Focal Chronic Pancreatitis and Pancreatic Adenocarcinoma

A CT examination is limited in identifying (early) ductal adenocarcinoma which begins during CP because of the reduced difference in density between the cancerous lesion, which is typically hypovascularized, and the pancreatic parenchyma, which is also hypovascularized due to the fibrosis. Furthermore, the main pancreatic duct, obstructed upstream by the lesion, already appears dilated due to the pre-existing chronic inflammatory processes. In rare cases, the onset of an adenocarcinoma in CP can sometimes be detected due to the displacement of ductal calcifications (Figure 4) with respect to previous CT examinations, indicating the presence of an expansive lesion.[114] Further, the presence of foci of calcification within the mass is believed to be a crucial radiologic criterion almost never seen in pancreatic duct adenocarcinoma.[115] This criterion only rarely is useful to aid in the differentiation between early CP and early pancreatic adenocarcinoma.

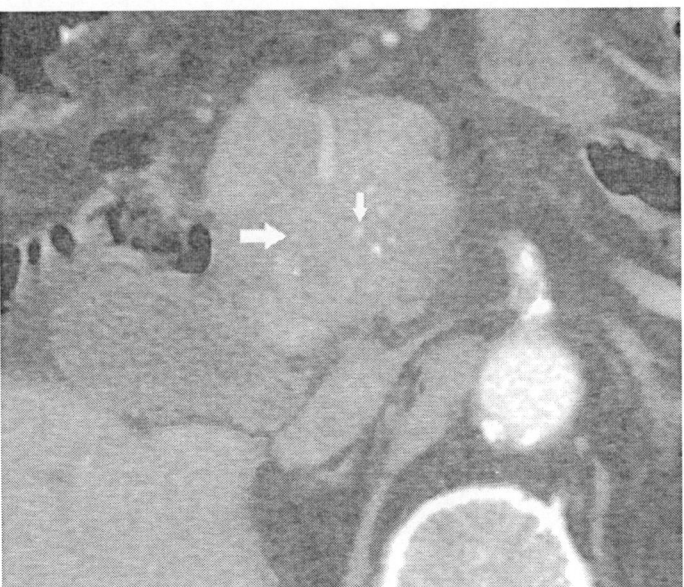

Figure 4a. CT-scan in the dynamic late arterial phase after IV injection of contrast agent displays an area of hypodensity (large white arrow) displacing some intrapancreatic calcifications. An underlying pancreatic cancer is likely in this case.

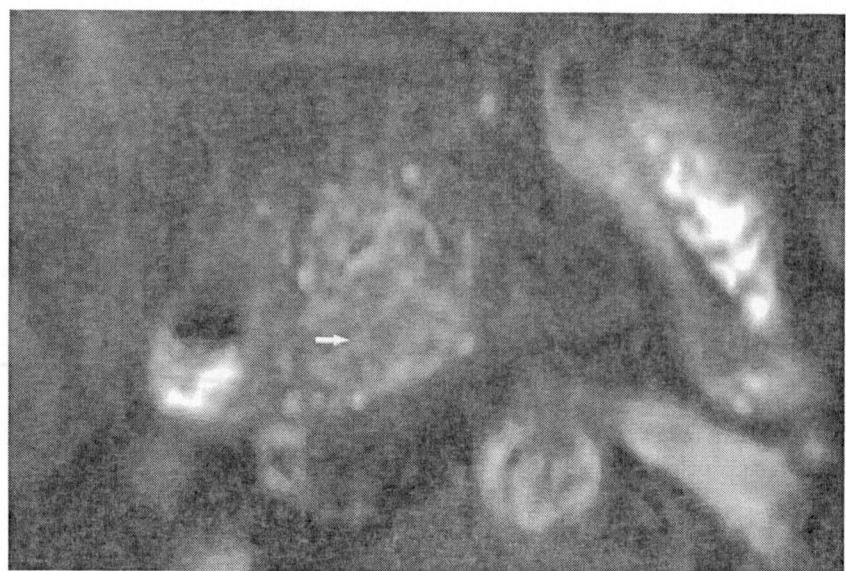

Figure 4b.

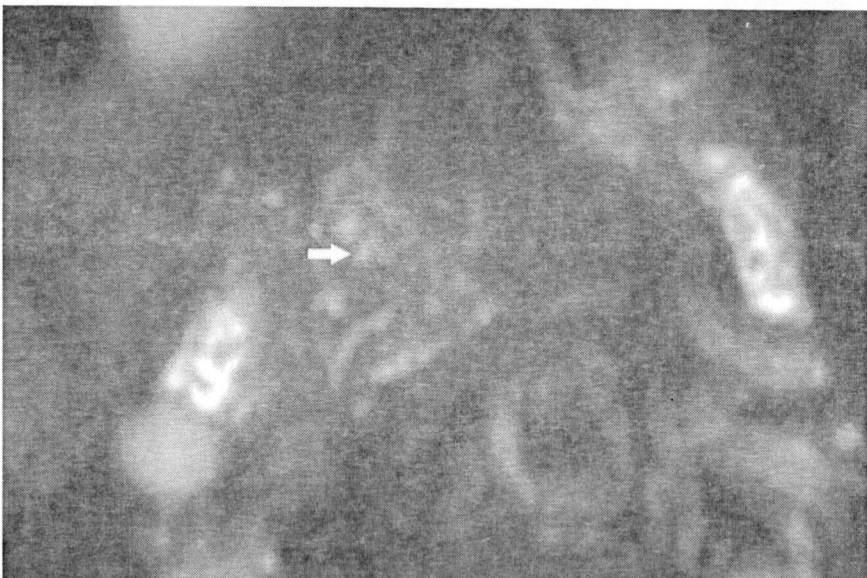

Figure 4c.

Figure 4b, 4c. T2w TSE (short TE) MRI-sequence in the transverse plane displays some dilated side branches ("duct-penetrating sign) in the pathologic area (white arrow).

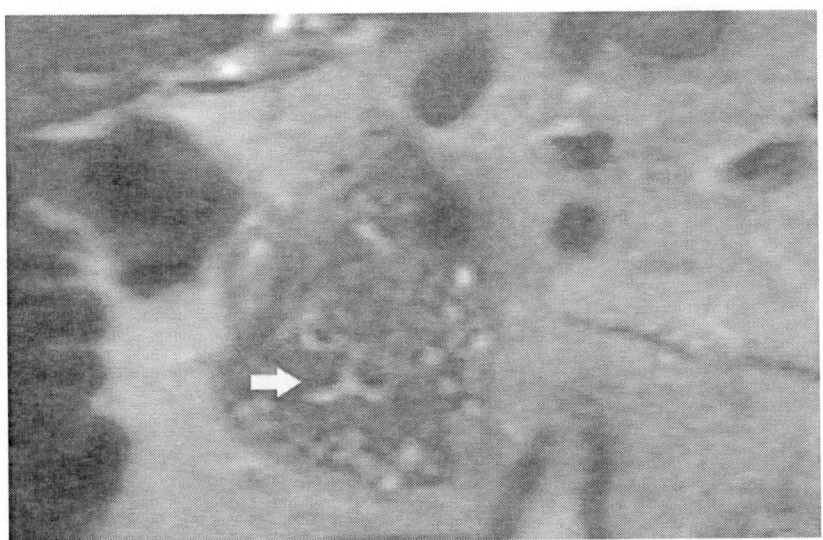

Figure 4d.

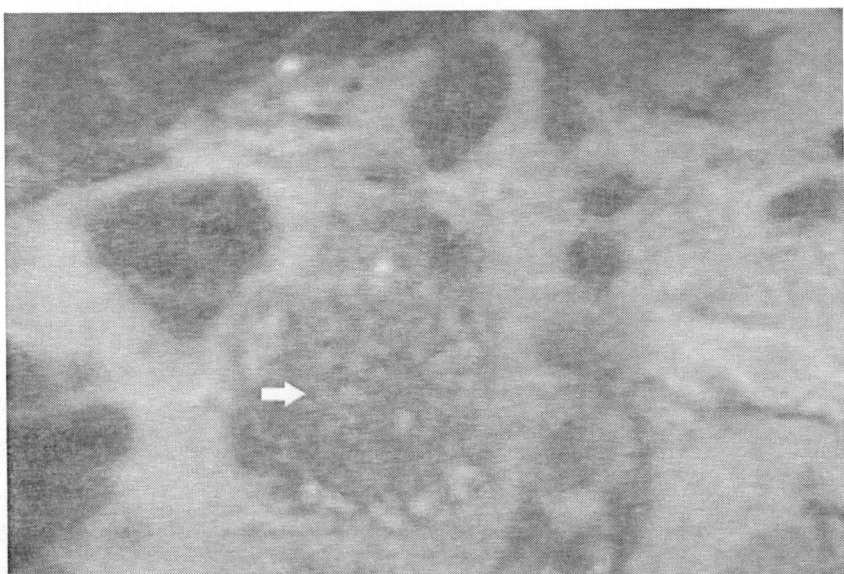

Figure 4e.

Figure 4d, 4e. T2w TSE (short TE) MRI-sequence in the coronal plane displays some dilated side branches ("duct-penetrating sign) in the pathologic area (white arrow).

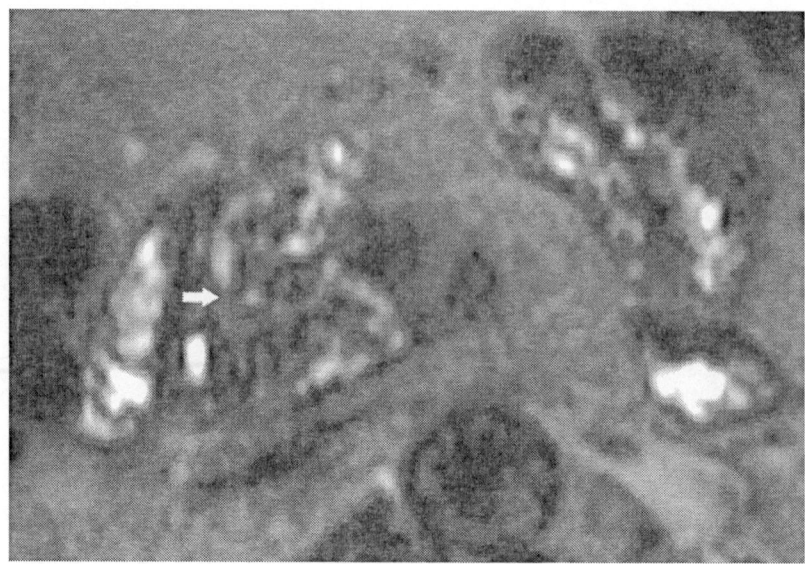

Figure 4f.

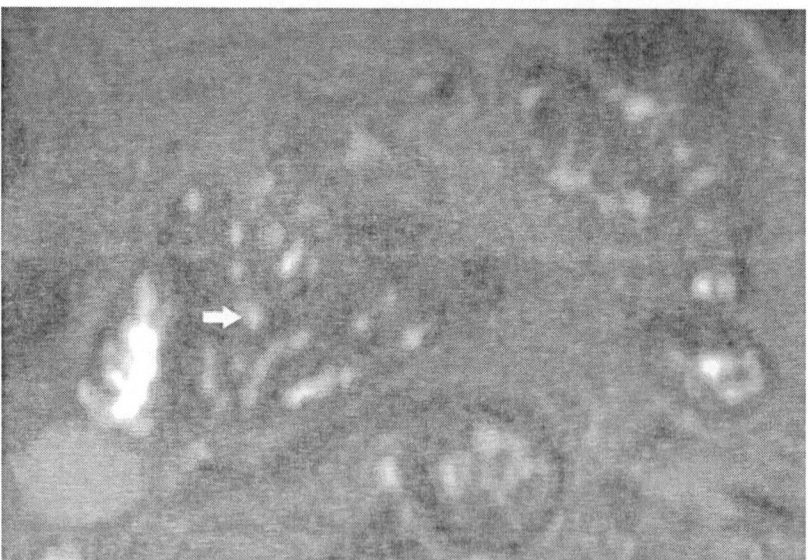

Figure 4g.

Figure 4f, 4g. T2w TSE (long TE) MRI-sequence in the transverse plane nicely displays some dilated side branches in the pathologic area (white arrow) indicative of the so-called "duct-penetrating" sign.

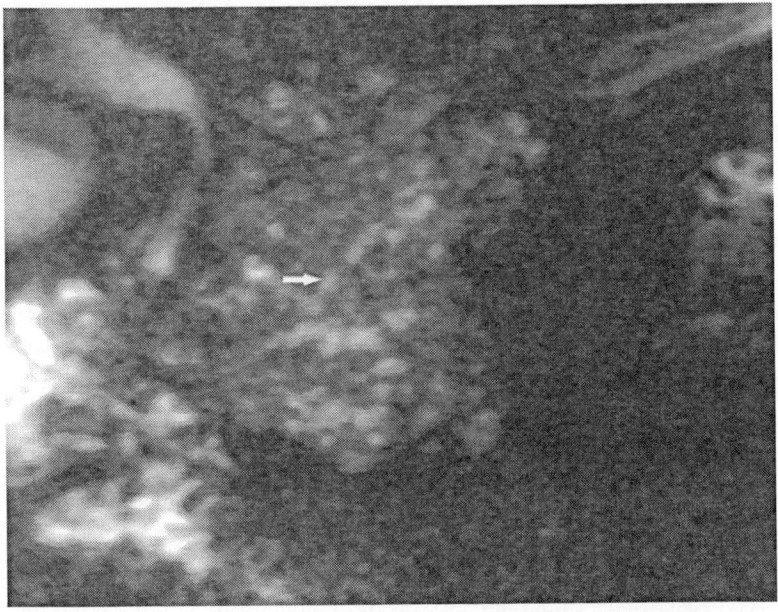

Figure 4h. MRCP-sequence again nicely displays some dilated side branches (white arrows) in the pathologic area. Also note the presence of a pancreatogram.

Magnetic Resonance Imaging in the Differentiation of Focal Chronic Pancreatitis and Pancreatic Adenocarcinoma

MRI is generally considered a valuable tool in the assessment of the full spectrum of pancreatic diseases. Relatively specific morphologic and signal intensity features permit characterization of CP and pancreatic duct adenocarcinoma in many cases but certainly not always. MRI studies can be considered in the following settings in patients with prior CT imaging who have focal enlargement of the pancreas with no definable mass or in patients in whom clinical history is worrisome for malignancy and in whom findings on CT imaging are equivocal or difficult to interpret and in situations requiring distinction between CP with focal enlargement and pancreatic cancer.[116] Still, differentiation between focal CP and a focal solid pancreatic cancer can be very difficult.

When findings of CP are identified in a patient without a prior history of CP or of ethanol abuse, an obstructing lesion should be suspected (Figure 5) [117].

Pancreatic duct adenocarcinoma is the usual cause of chronic obstructive pancreatitis and comprises 75% to 90% of all pancreatic adenocarcinomas (Figure 6).[118] Differentiating between an inflammatory mass due to CP and pancreatic adenocarcinoma on the basis of imaging criteria remains difficult. Irregularity of the pancreatic duct, intraductal or parenchymal calcifications, diffuse pancreatic involvement, and normal or smoothly stenotic pancreatic duct penetrating through the mass ("duct penetrating sign") favor the diagnosis of CP over pancreatic adenocarcinoma (Figure 7, Figure 8).[110] In distinction, a smoothly dilated pancreatic duct with an abrupt interruption, dilatation of both biliary and pancreatic ducts ("double-duct sign"), and obliteration of the perivascular fat planes favor the diagnosis of cancer. MRI may be superior to CT for the evaluation of pancreatic adenocarcinoma, especially if the lesion is small and non-contour-deforming. The tumor is often best delineated on unenhanced T1w FS images and multiphasic contrast-enhanced sequences [32]. However, as mentioned, even when using MRI, differentiating (early) pancreatic adenocarcinoma from mass-forming focal CP remains difficult. Typically, the chronically inflamed pancreas will enhance more than will pancreatic adenocarcinoma on immediate postgadolinium images, particularly those tumors arising in the head. Unfortunately, the degree of contrast-enhancement cannot be used to reliably distinguish these entities because abundant fibrosis is seen in both CP and adenocarcinoma, accounting for their similar appearances [110].

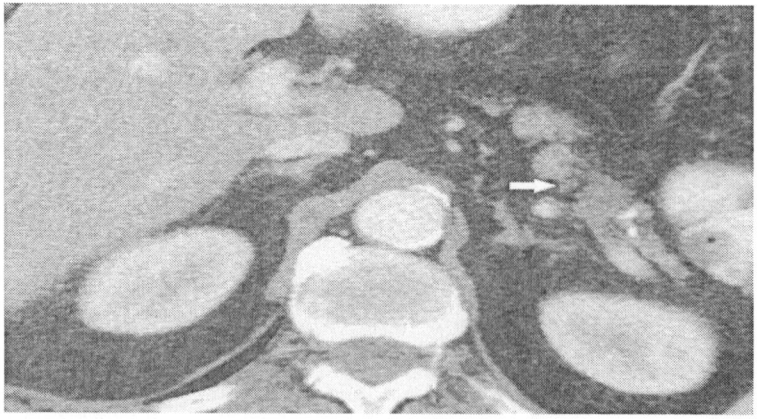

Figure 5a. CT-scan in a delayed venous phase (2 minutes post IV injection of contrast agent) displaying a persisting hypodense area (white arrow) at the level of the pancreatic tail. More proximally, the pancreatic tail shows signs of hypodensity caused by obstructive inflammation of the pancreatic parenchyma.

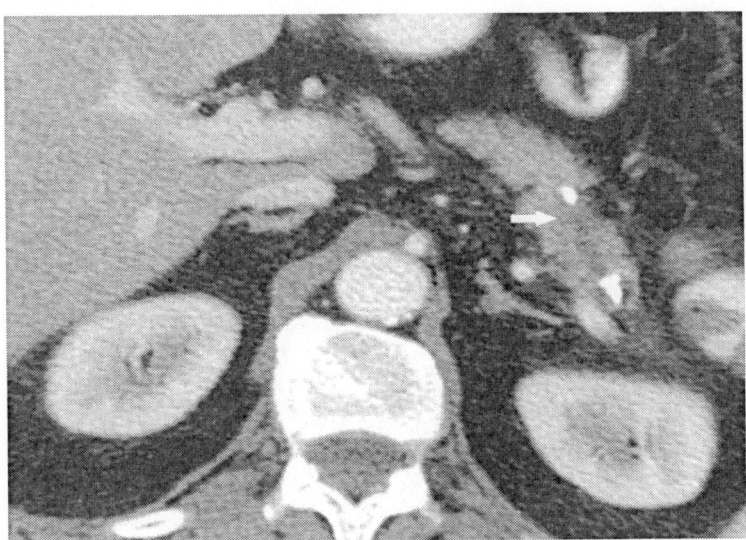

Figure 5b. CT-scan in a delayed venous phase (2 minutes post IV injection of contrast agent) displaying the earlier mentioned persisting hypodense area (white arrow) and some nearby calcifications at the level of the pancreatic tail.

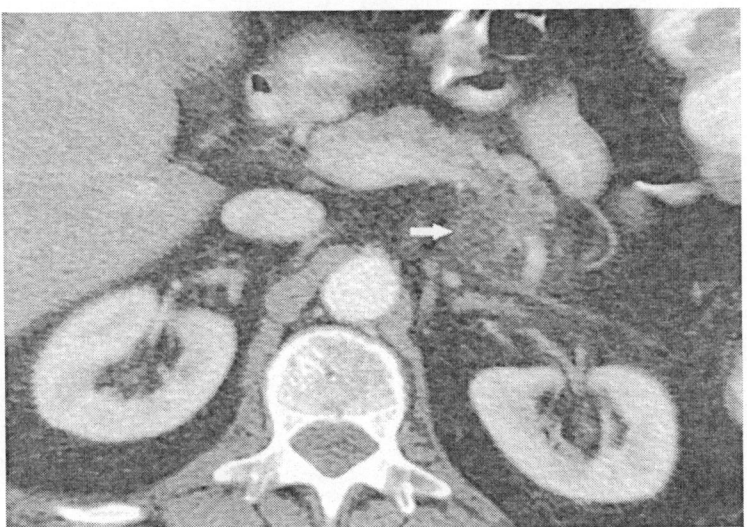

Figure 5c. CT-scan in a delayed venous phase (2 minutes post IV injection of contrast agent) displaying the earlier mentioned persisting hypodense area (white arrow) associated with an area of focal inflammation of the peripancreatic fatty tissue.

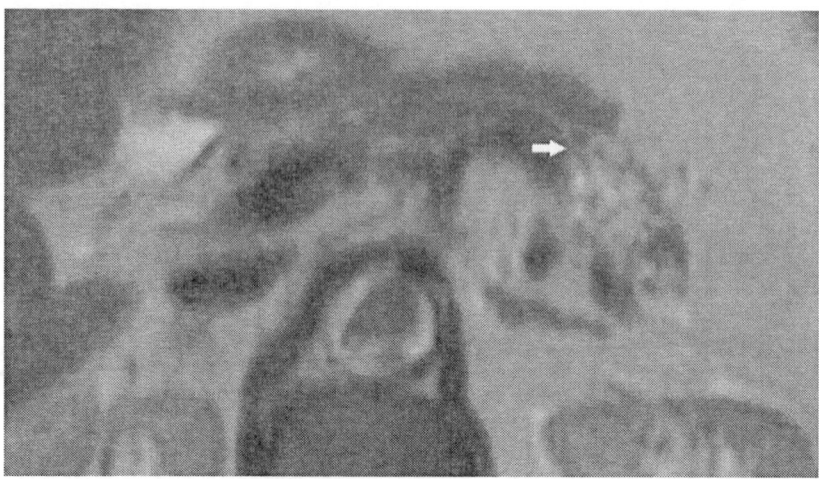

Figure 5d. T2w TSE (short TE) MRI-sequence displaying a clearly distinctive border (white arrow) between normal and pathologic (proximal part of pancreatic tail) pancreatic parenchyma. The pathologic pancreatic parenchyma is clearly more hyperintense due to edema at some dilated side branches at this level.

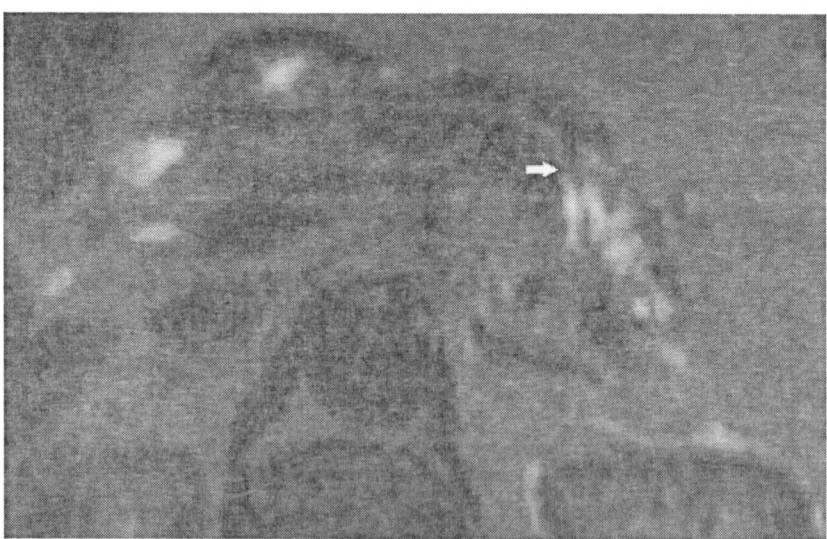

Figure 5e. T2w TSE (long TE) MRI-sequence displaying the above mentioned clearly distinctive border (white arrow) between normal and pathologic (proximal part of pancreatic tail) pancreatic parenchyma. The pathologic pancreatic parenchyma is clearly more hyperintense due to edema at some dilated side branches at this level.

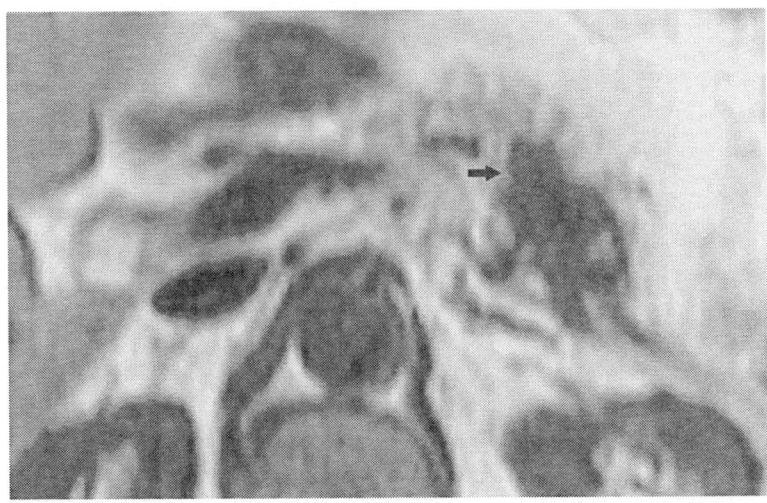

Figure 5f. T1w GE MRI-sequence before IV injection of contrast agent and without fat suppression also displays the above mentioned clearly distinctive border (black arrow) between normal and pathologic (proximal part of pancreatic tail) pancreatic parenchyma. The pathologic pancreatic parenchyma is clearly more hypointense on T1w imaging due to edema and decrease of protein-rich pancreatic juice. The normal part of the pancreatic parenchyma is clearly hyperintense due to the high protein concentration of the pancreatic juice.

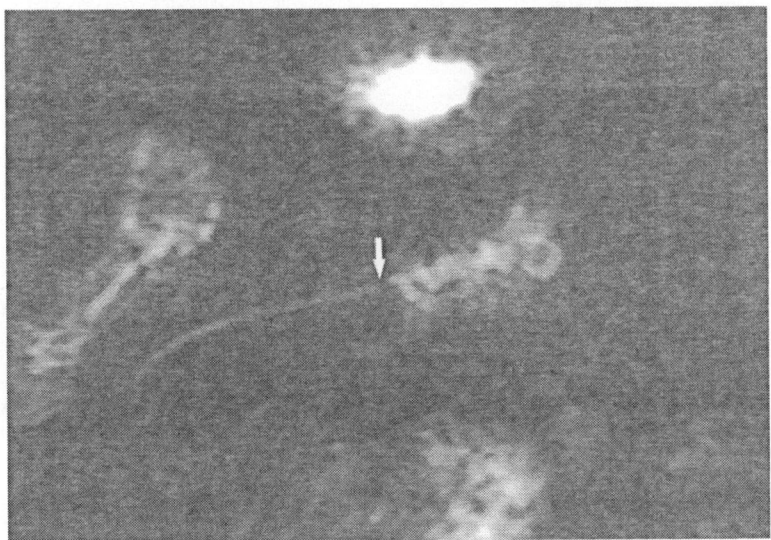

Figure 5g.

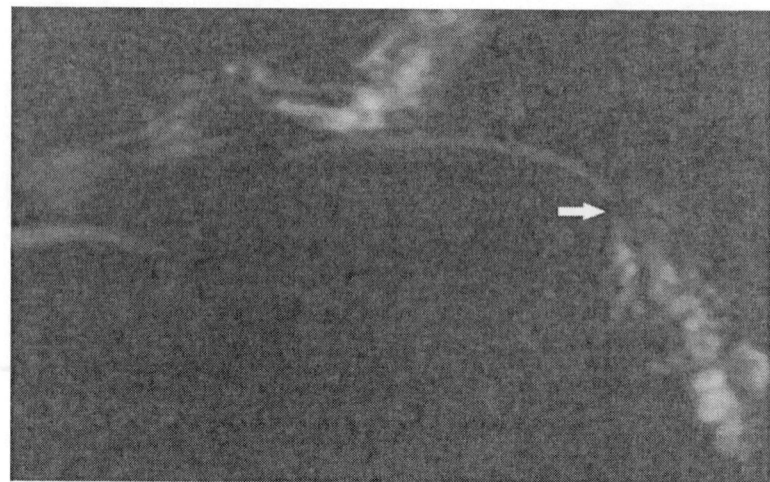

Figure 5h.

Figure 5g, 5h. MRCP-sequence again displaying a clearly distinctive border (white arrow) between normal and pathologic (proximal part of pancreatic tail) pancreatic parenchyma. The pathologic pancreatic parenchyma is clearly more hyperintense due to edema at some dilated side branches at this level. Also notice a focal distinctive narrowing of the main pancreatic duct (white arrow) necessitating the search for or the exclusion of a focal pancreatic cancer.

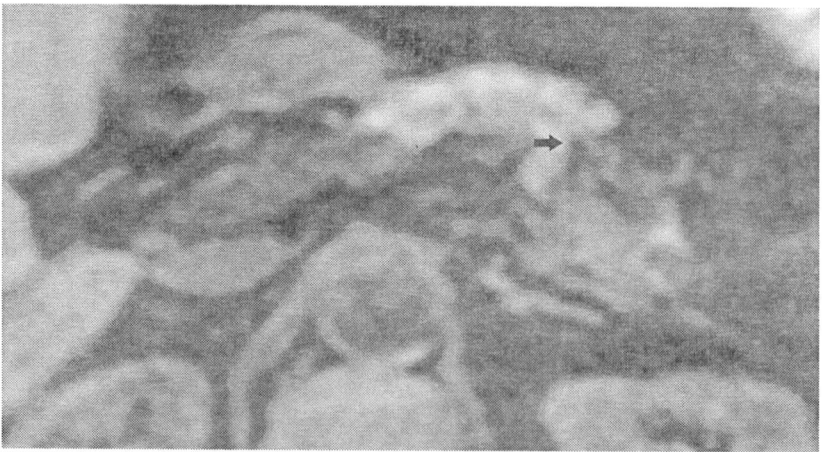

Figure 5i. T1w GE MRI-sequence with fat suppression before IV injection of contrast agent displaying the above mentioned clearly distinctive border (black arrow) between normal and pathologic (proximal part of pancreatic tail) pancreatic parenchyma.

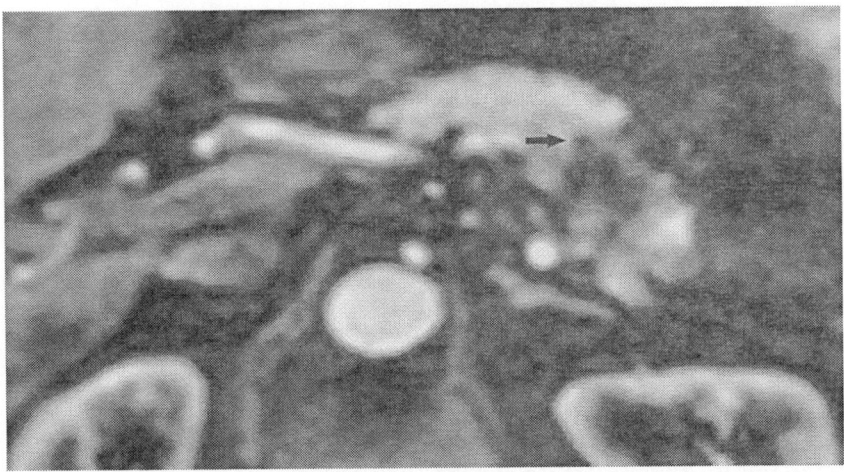

Figure 5j. T1w GE MRI-sequence with fat suppression in the dynamic late arterial phase after IV injection of contrast agent displaying the above mentioned clearly distinctive border (black arrow) between normal and pathologic (proximal part of pancreatic tail) pancreatic parenchyma. The pathologic pancreatic parenchyma is clearly less contrast-enhancing when compared with the normal pancreatic parenchyma.

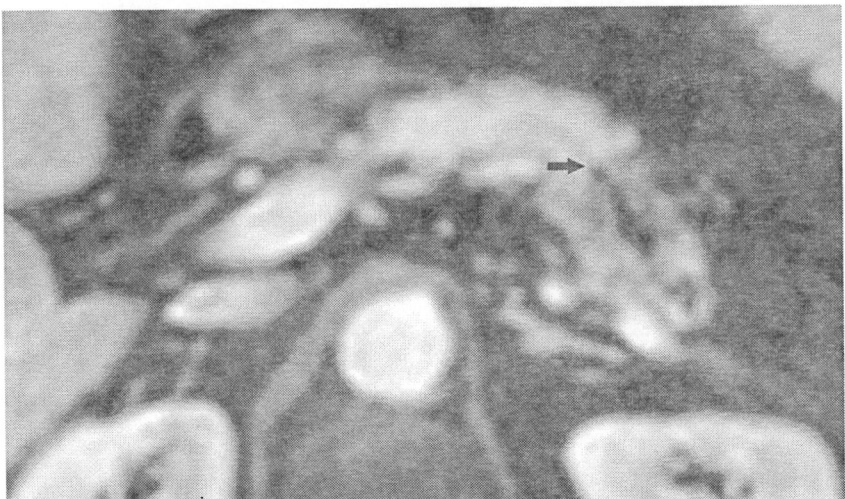

Figure 5k. T1w GE MRI-sequence with fat suppression in the early venous phase after IV injection of contrast agent displaying the above mentioned clearly distinctive border (black arrow) between normal and pathologic (proximal part of pancreatic tail) pancreatic parenchyma. The pathologic pancreatic parenchyma is clearly less contrast-enhancing when compared with the normal pancreatic parenchyma.

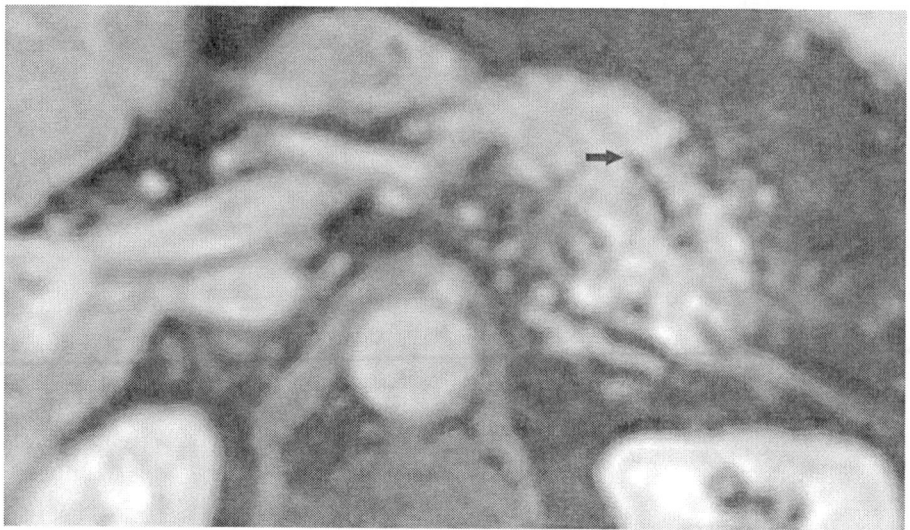

Figure 51. T1w GE MRI-sequence with fat suppression in the delayed venous phase 5 minutes after IV injection of contrast agent. The border (black arrow) between normal and pathologic (proximal part of pancreatic tail) pancreatic parenchyma is hard to discriminate. This border can mainly be detected by an abrupt narrowing of the main pancreatic duct (black arrow) at this level. No underlying pancreatic cancer/solid mass can be detected.

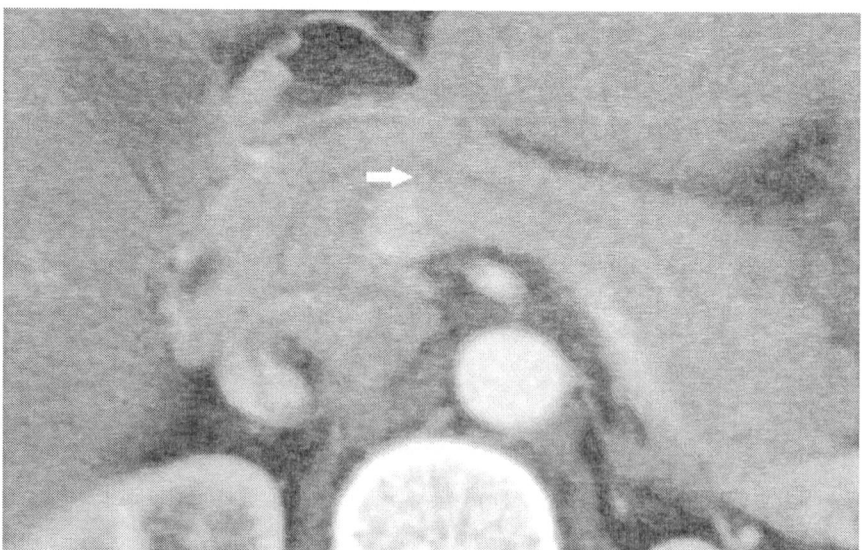

Figure 6a.

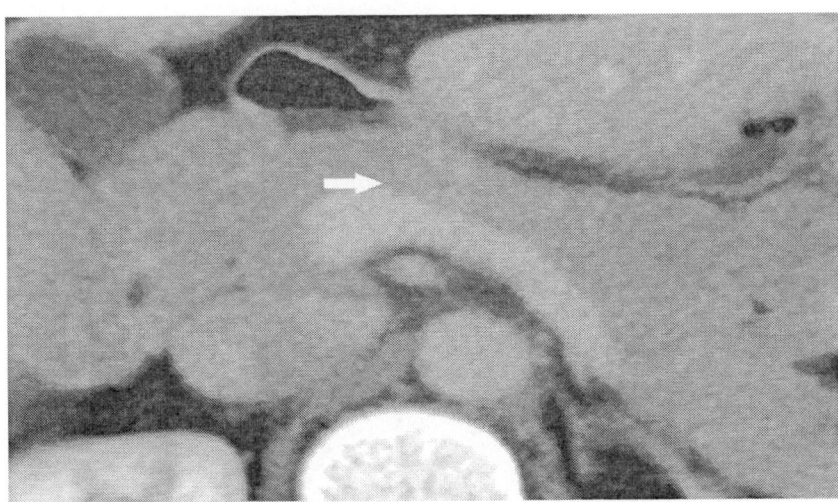

Figure 6b.

Figure 6a, 6b. CT-scan in the dynamic late arterial phase after IV injection of contrast agent displaying an enlarged main pancreatic duct. No solid mass is seen at the level of the white arrow.

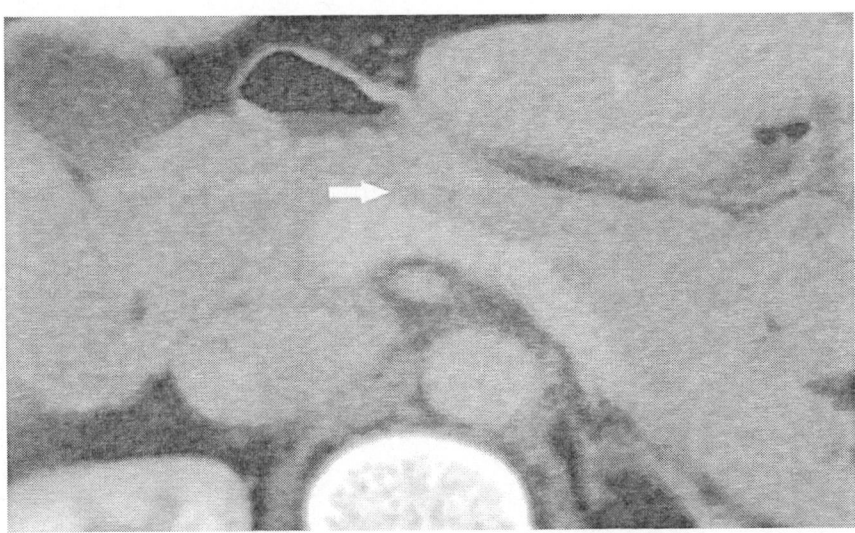

Figure 6c. BlackBlood Single Shot Spin Echo Echo Planar Imaging (BB SS SE-EPI) using a low diffusion gradient ($b=10s/mm^2$) in the transverse plane clearly displays one focal hyperintensity (white arrow) at the level of the pancreatic body. This finding is very suggestive of an underlying solid mass.

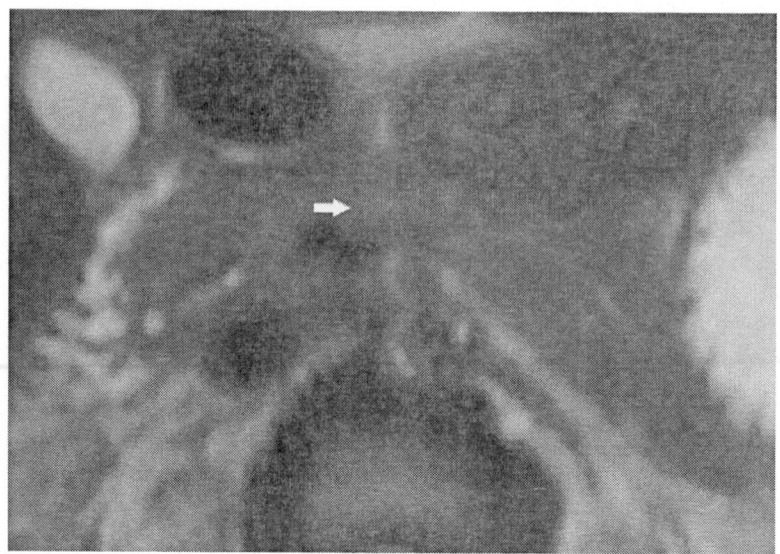

Figure 6d. T2w TSE (short TE) MRI-sequence in the transverse plane displaying an enlarged main pancreatic duct. A slight hyperintense area might be identified retrospectively.

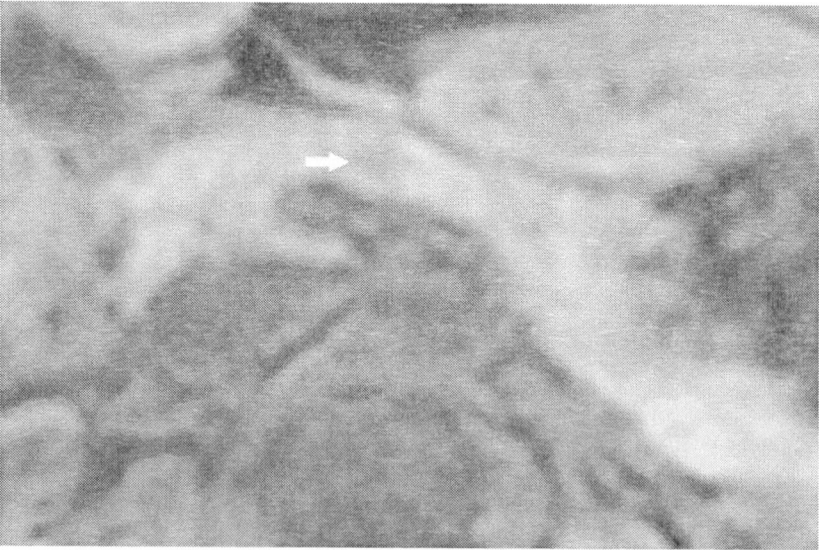

Figure 6e. T1w GE MRI-sequence before IV injection of contrast agent and with fat suppression displays a discrete hypointensity (white arrow) at the level of the pancreatic body.

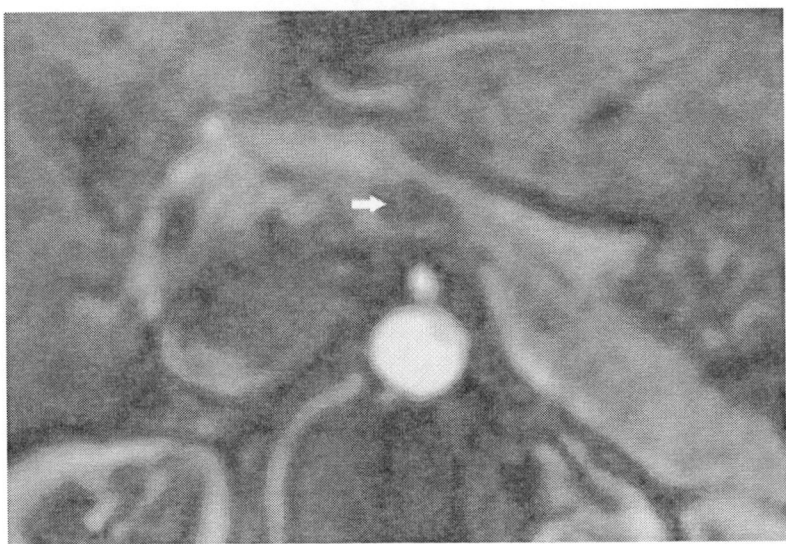

Figure 6f. T1w GE MRI-sequence with fat suppression in the dynamic late arterial phase after IV injection of contrast agent displays the above mentioned hypointensity (white arrow) more clearly.

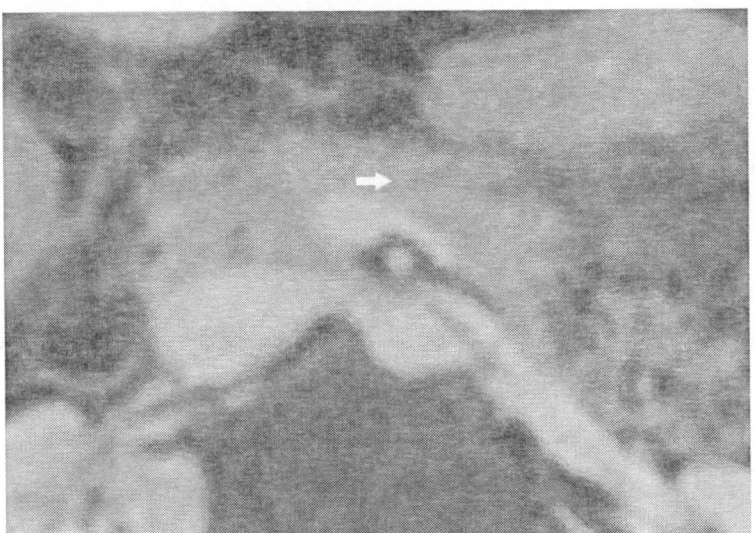

Figure 6g. T1w GE MRI-sequence with fat suppression in the delayed venous phase 5 minutes after IV injection of contrast agent displays the above mentioned hypointensity (white arrow) less clearly. This finding is rather suggestive for chronic pancreatitis.

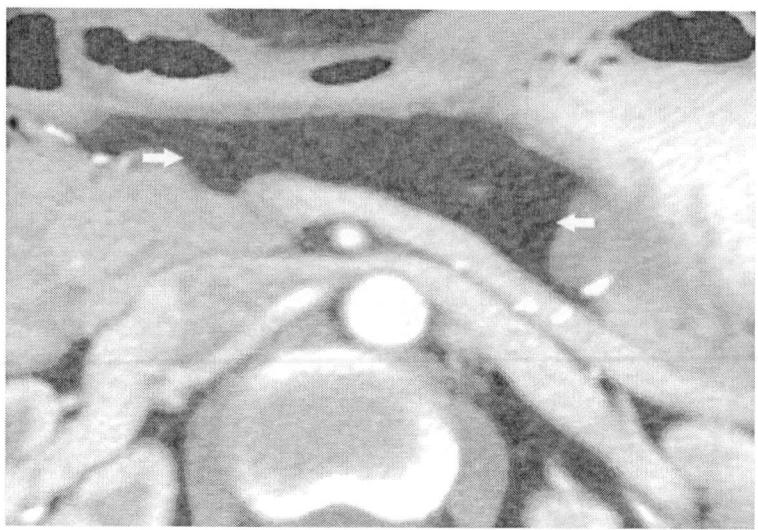

Figure 6h. CT-scan in the dynamic late arterial phase after IV injection of contrast agent displaying the remaining pancreatic parenchyma post-resection. A small focal pancreatic cancer was confirmed histopathologically.

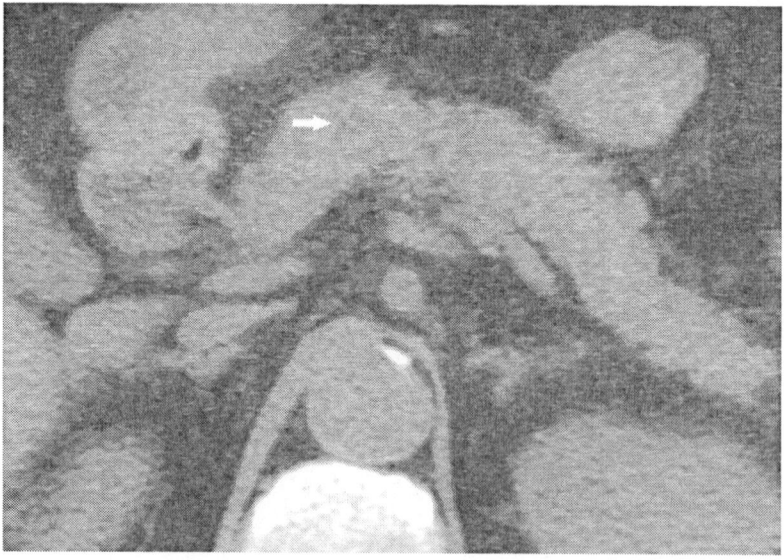

Figure 7a. CT-scan before IV injection of contrast agent displaying a discrete hypodense area (white arrow) at the level of the pancreatic neck. No further signs of pathology are seen.

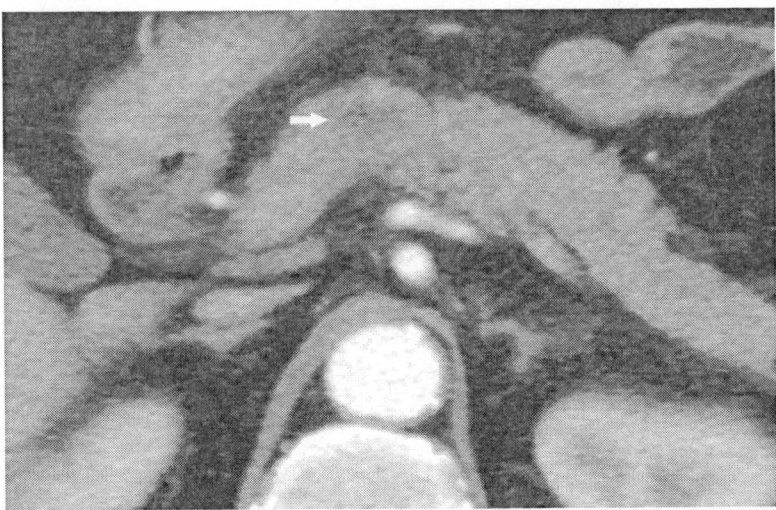

Figure 7b. CT-scan in the dynamic late arterial phase after IV injection of contrast agent more clearly displaying the above mentioned hypodense area (white arrow) at the level of the pancreatic neck. No further signs of pathology are seen.

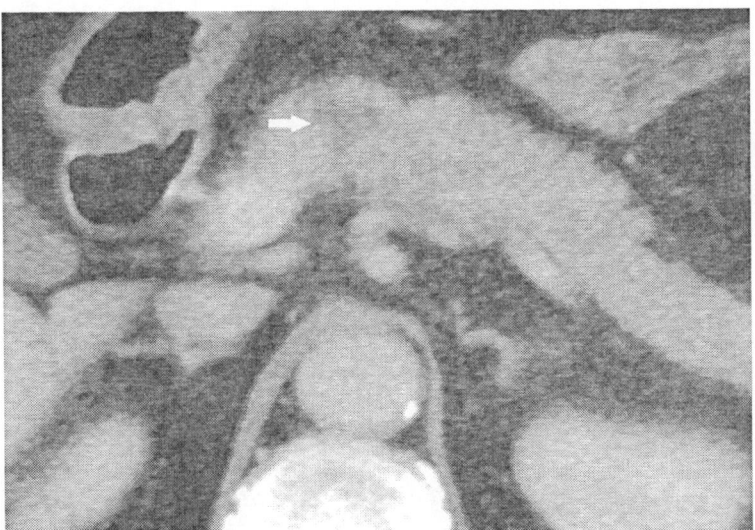

Figure 7c. CT-scan in the dynamic early venous phase after IV injection of contrast agent clearly displaying the above mentioned hypodense area (white arrow) at the level of the pancreatic neck. No further signs of pathology are seen. Using CT-scan in this case, the differential diagnosis between focal chronic pancreatitis and focal pancreatic cancer was very difficult.

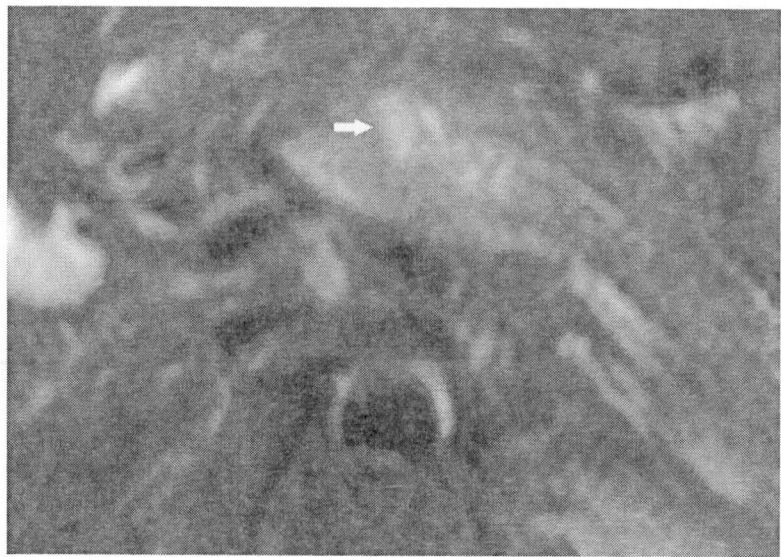

Figure 7d. T2w TSE (short TE) MRI-sequence displaying a moderate to frank hyperintense area (white arrow) at the level of the pancreatic neck. An abutting pathologically dilated side branch, indicative for chronic pancreatitis, is also depicted.

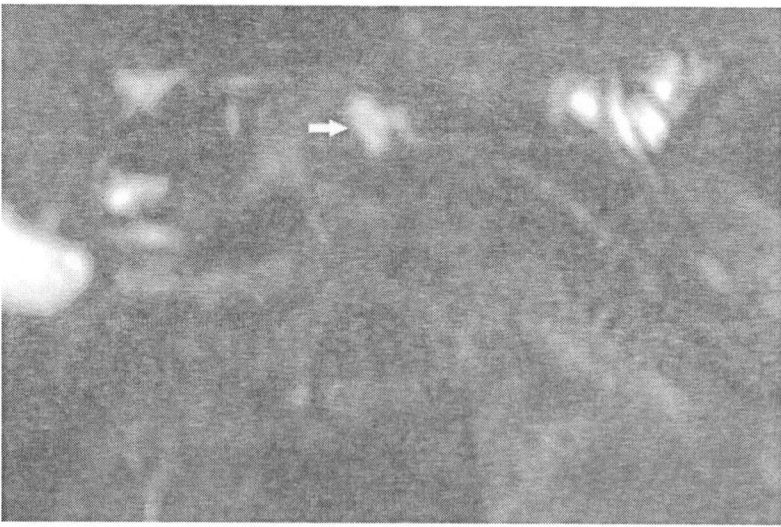

Figure 7e. T2w TSE (long TE) MRI-sequence still displaying the above mentioned area as hyperintense (white arrow) indicative for fluid (cyst). An abutting pathologically dilated side branch, indicative for chronic pancreatitis, is also depicted.

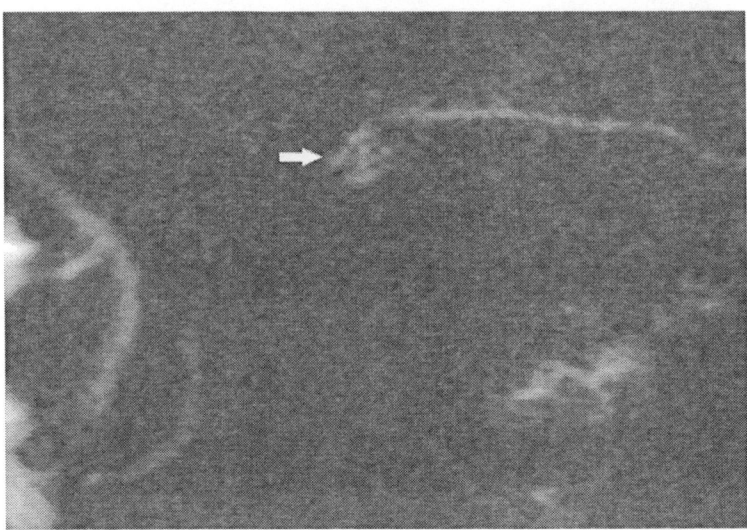

Figure 7f. MRCP-sequence displaying the above mentioned area as hyperintense (white arrow). An abutting pathologically dilated side branch, indicative for chronic pancreatitis, is also depicted.

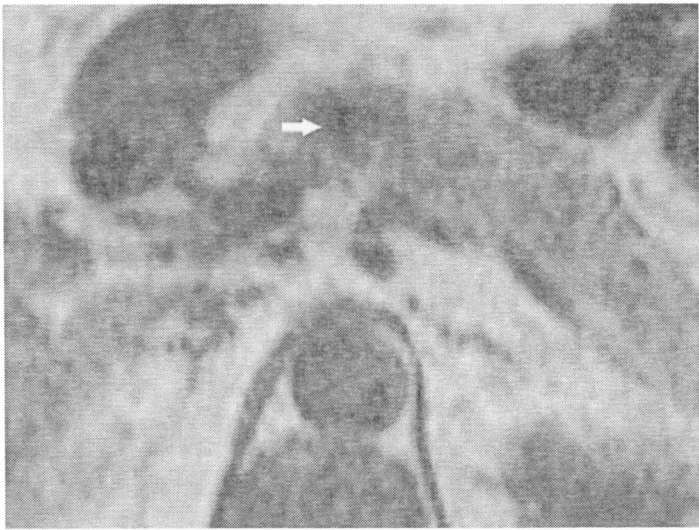

Figure 7g. T1w GE MRI-sequence before IV injection of contrast agent and without fat suppression displays the above mentioned area as hypointense (white arrow). Furthermore, the signal intensity of the remaining pancreatic parenchyma is too low, suggestive of pancreatitis.

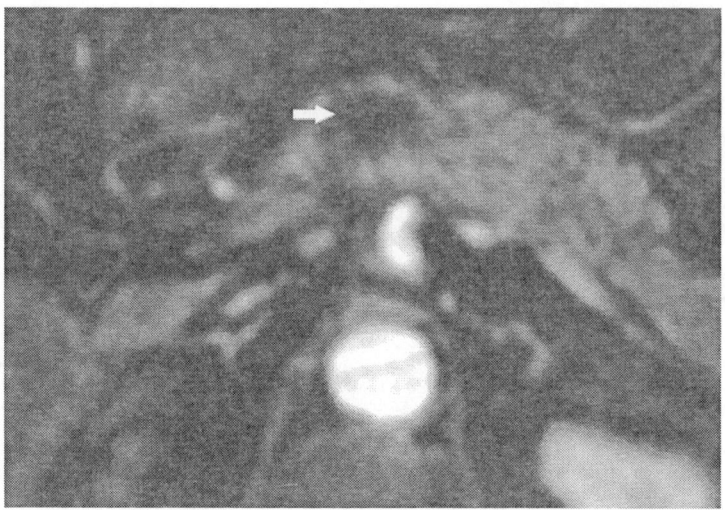

Figure 7h. T1w GE MRI-sequence with fat suppression in the dynamic late arterial phase after IV injection of contrast agent displaying the above mentioned area as hypointense (white arrow). No contrast-enhancement is seen at this level. The remaining pancreatic parenchyma displays heterogenous contrast-enhancement.

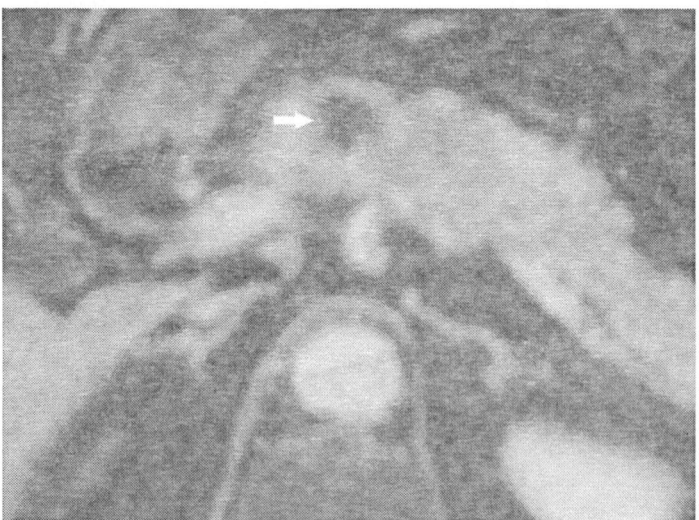

Figure 7i. T1w GE MRI-sequence with fat suppression in the delayed venous phase 5 minutes after IV injection of contrast agent displaying the above mentioned area as hypointense (white arrow). No contrast-enhancement is seen at this level. The remaining pancreatic parenchyma displays heterogenous contrast-enhancement.

A study of Kim T. et al. [119] revealed two different enhancement patterns in pancreatic masses due to focal CP as seen on two-phase helical CT and on dynamic MRI: pancreatic masses due to CP appeared as hypoenhanced demarcated masses or as isoenhancing nondemarcated masses on pancreatic phase images. The two different enhancement patterns in masses due to CP might be explained by the difference in the degree of fibrosis between the mass and the nonenlarged portion of the pancreas. Fibrosis was pathologically identified in the nonenlarged portion of the pancreas in patients with nondemarcated masses on CT scans or MRI images, whereas fibrosis was not found in the nonenlarged portion of the pancreas in patients with demarcated masses. Fibrosis is one of the main pathologic changes characteristic of CP.[2] Therefore, when CP occurs focally, the inflammatory mass is visibly demarcated on CT scans or on MRI images.

On the other hand, when CP occurs throughout the pancreas, the mass is not demarcated. It is thought that the hypoenhanced and demarcated pancreatic mass due to CP on pancreatic phase contrast-enhanced helical CT or MRI is not distinguishable from pancreatic adenocarcinoma, whereas the isoenhanced and nondemarcated masses may be distinguishable from hypovascular pancreatic adenocarcinoma or other hypervascular pancreatic tumors. However, histologic examination or close interval follow-up is needed for such isoenhanced and nondemarcated pancreatic masses. Tumor-free pancreatic parenchyma located proximally to a pancreatic adenocarcinoma obstructing the pancreatic duct may undergo atrophy and fibrosis and thus may show the same gradual enhancement pattern as pancreatic adenocarcinoma [110], whereas pancreatic adenocarcinoma located in the pancreatic head may show isoenhancement and no demarcation. In their study, two different enhancement patterns on two-phase helical CT and dynamic MRI were identified in masses due to CP. When histologic fibrosis is uniformly present through the gland in patients with CP, there is no demarcation of masses due to CP. When there is a greater degree of histologic fibrosis in the masslike part of the gland, the mass is often demarcated from the remaining pancreas, and the enhancement pattern on two-phase helical CT and dynamic gadolinium-enhanced MRI mimics that of pancreatic adenocarcinoma. Further work is needed to improve the rate of correct diagnosis of masses due to focal CP. Following our own experience, unenhanced T1w GE FS sequence (in combination with T2w imaging) often is a very accurate radiologic sequence allowing to detect a focal pancreatic adenocarcinoma appearing more hypointense compared with the surrounding pancreatic parenchyma (even in the presence of more proximally located obstructive CP). Comparable findings were published by Sica GT et al. using unenhanced T1w FS spin-echo [64].

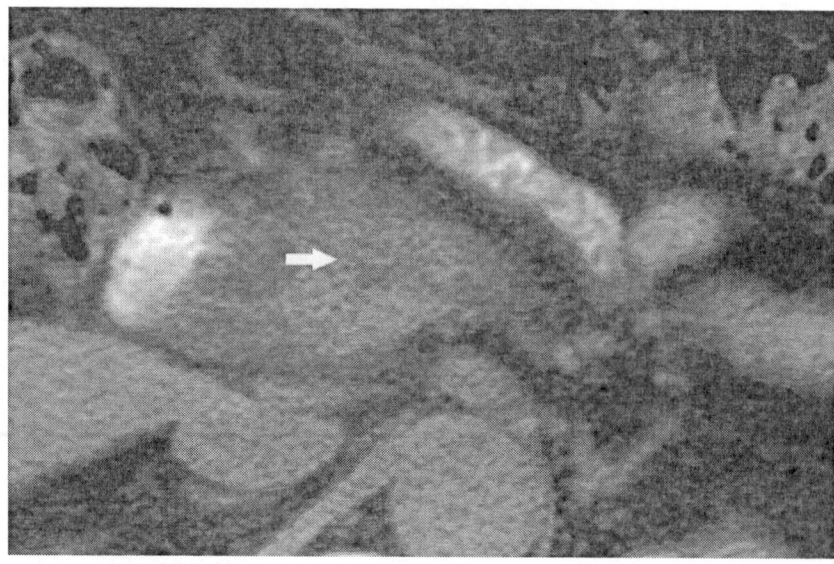

Figure 8a. CT-scan before IV injection of contrast agent displaying a hypodense area (white arrow) at the level of the pancreatic head.

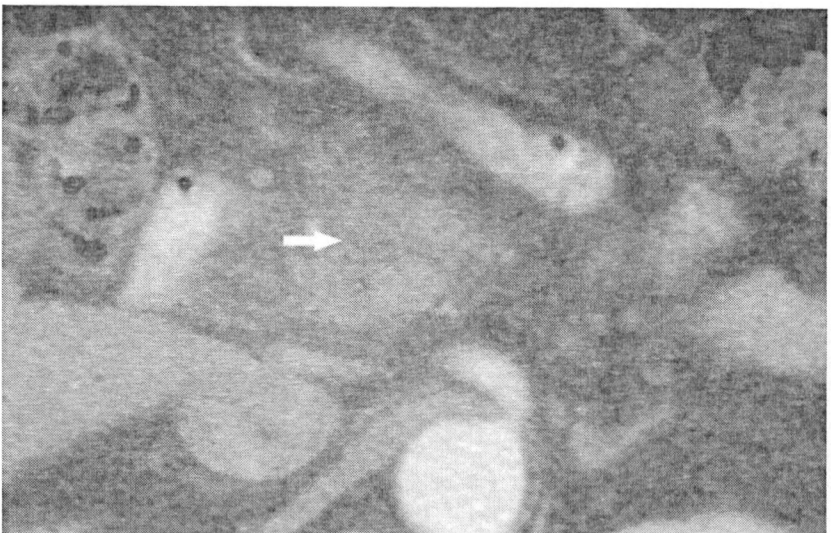

Figure 8b. CT-scan in the dynamic late arterial phase after IV injection of contrast agent more clearly displaying the above mentioned hypodense area (white arrow) at the level of the pancreatic head. Infiltration of the surrounding pancreatic fatty tissue is seen.

Differentiation of an Early Neoplastic and Inflammatory Mass... 49

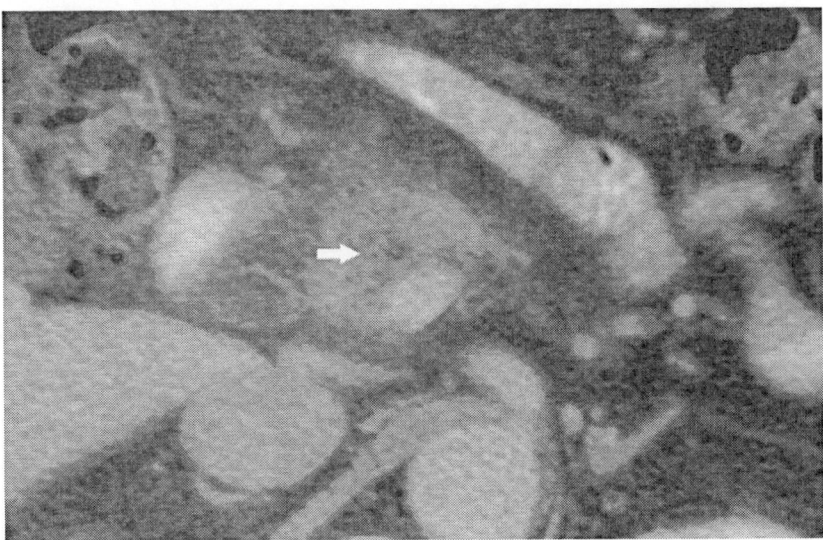

Figure 8c. CT-scan in the dynamic early venous phase after IV injection of contrast agent clearly displaying the above mentioned hypodense area (white arrow) at the level of the pancreatic head. An atypical hypodensity is seen in the center of this area.

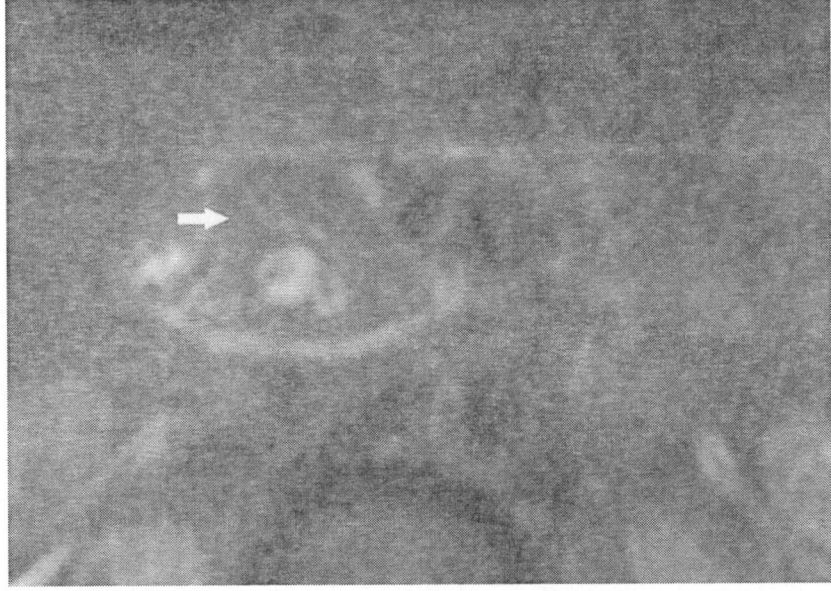

Figure 8d.

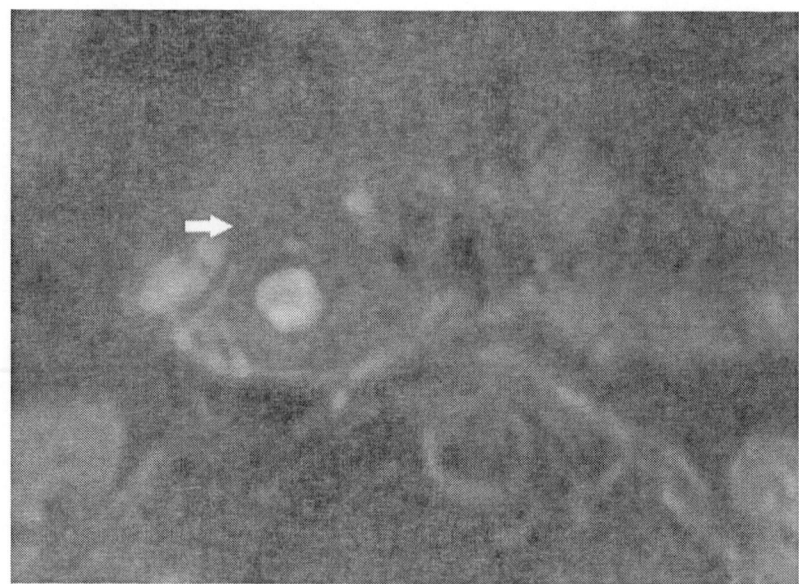

Figure 8e.

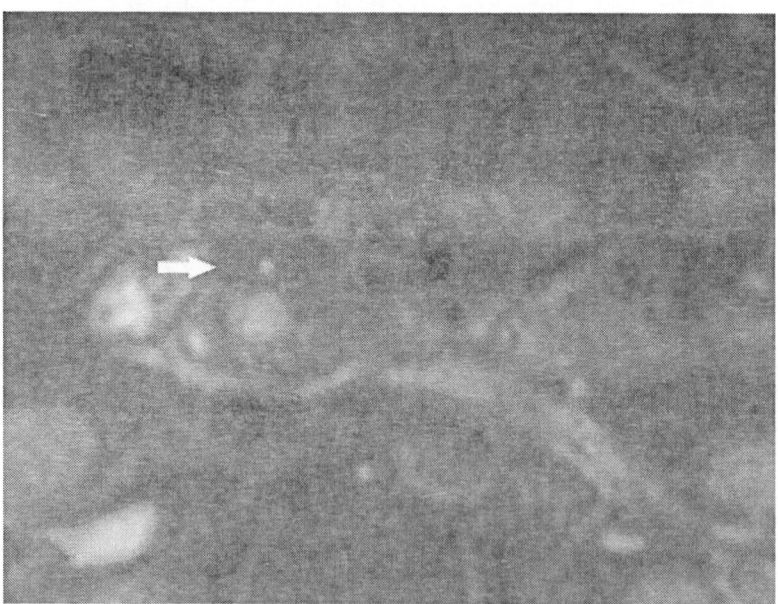

Figure 8f.

Figure 8d, 8e, 8f. T2w TSE (long TE) MRI-sequence in the transverse plane displays a dilated side branch ("duct-penetrating" sign) in the pathologic area (white arrow).

Differentiation of an Early Neoplastic and Inflammatory Mass... 51

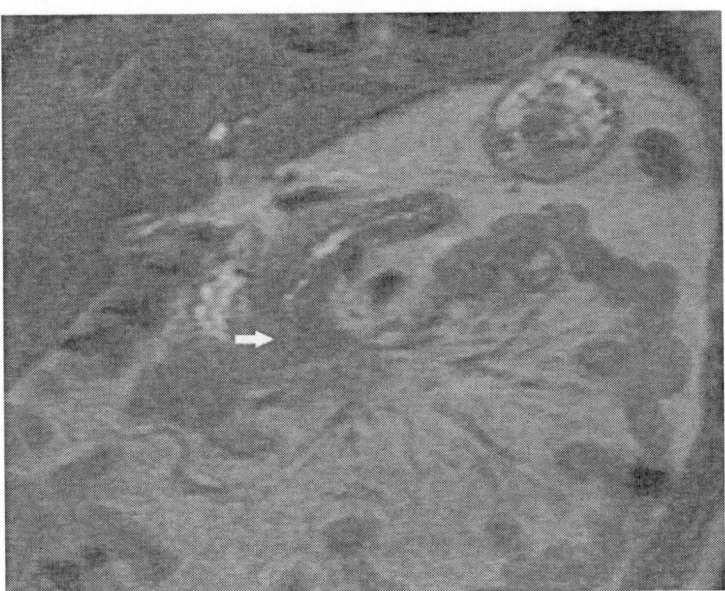

Figure 8g. T2w TSE (long TE) MRI-sequence in the coronal plane nicely displays some dilated side branches in the pathologic area (white arrow) indicative of the so-called "duct-penetrating" sign.

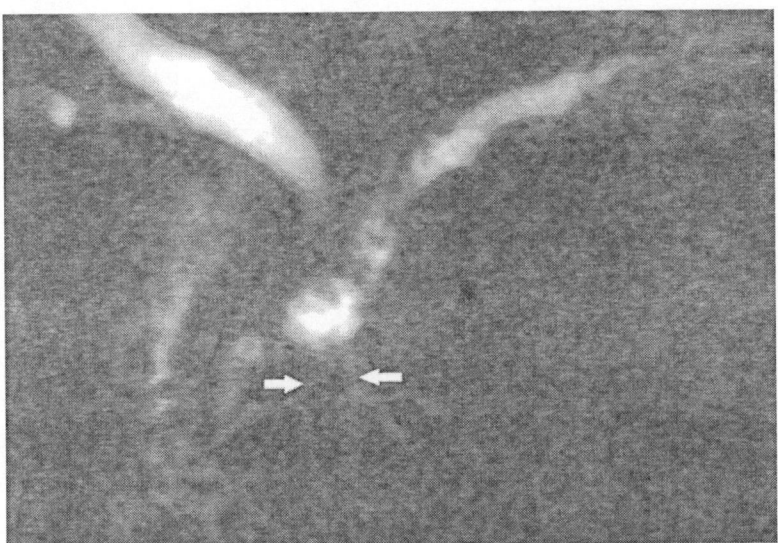

Figure 8h. MRCP-sequence again nicely displays some dilated side branches (white arrows) in the pathologic area.

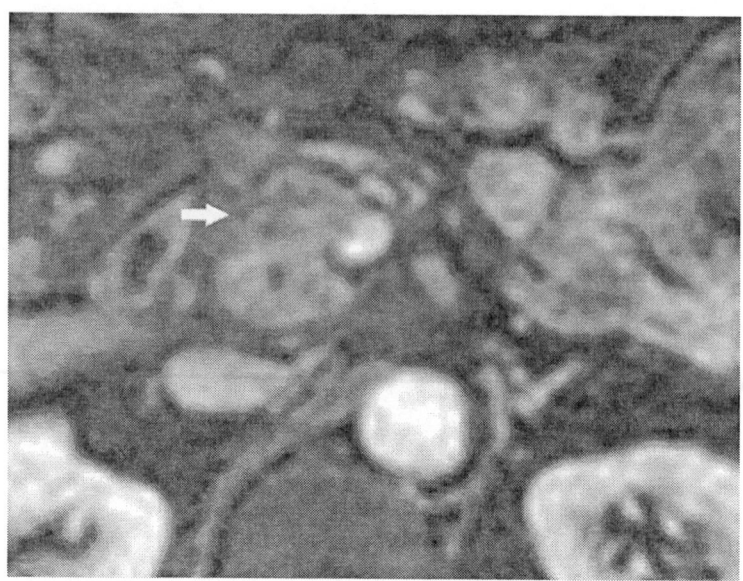

Figure 8i. T1w GE MRI-sequence with fat suppression in the delayed venous phase 5 minutes after IV injection of contrast agent displaying the above mentioned area as hypointense (white arrow). In this case, the diagnosis of focal chronic pancreatitis rather than pancreatic cancer is mainly made on the basis of the T2w sequences ("duct-penetrating" sign). T1w sequences were not useful in this case.

MRCP may be helpful to aid in this differentiation, because chronic alcoholic pancreatitis, compared with chronic obstructive pancreatitis due to adenocarcinoma, is more frequently associated with an irregularly dilated duct with intraductal calcification.[120] The ratio of duct caliber to pancreatic gland width is higher in patients with adenocarcinoma.[121] Also, the "duct-penetrating sign," seen in 85% of CP and in only 4% of patients with cancer, helps to distinguish an inflammatory pancreatic mass from pancreatic adenocarcinoma. The "duct-penetrating sign" refers to a non-obstructed main pancreatic duct penetrating an inflammatory pancreatic mass, unlike its usual obstruction by pancreatic adenocarcinoma.[122] Furthermore, MRCP can depict the classic "double-duct sign" of pancreatic adenocarcinoma (enlargement and non-communication of the pancreatic and common bile ducts).[123] A normal-sized pancreatic duct is present in up to 20% of patients with adenocarcinoma, however, and should not dissuade its diagnosis in the setting of common bile duct dilation. MRI detection of early pancreatic cancer without pancreatic duct involvement has not been adequately studied [124].

Positron Emission Tomography in the Differentiation of Focal Chronic Pancreatitis and Pancreatic Adenocarcinoma

Positron Emission Tomography (PET) with 2-fluoro-2-deoxy-D-glucose (FDG) was recently introduced into clinical oncology because of its ability to demonstrate metabolic changes associated with various disease processes. Some studies investigated the possibility of identifying pancreatic cancer in CP with FDG-PET. [125, 126]

Tissue Diagnosis in the Differentiation of Focal Chronic Pancreatitis and Pancreatic Adenocarcinoma

Tissue diagnosis (cytologic or histologic examination) is mostly performed in the differential diagnosis between focal CP and pancreatic cancer. EUS-FNA is becoming the standard for obtaining cytologic diagnosis, although the sensitivity of EUS-FNA for the differential diagnosis of pancreatic masses is variable in the literature, being as low as 75% in some studies.[105] Moreover, the sensitivity was reported to be unacceptably lower (54%) in the context of CP, whereas surgical resection was still necessary to confirm the diagnosis.[106] Consequently, EUS-FNA in patients with pancreatic masses has a low negative predictive value, and its ability to differentiate between pancreatic cancer and pseudotumoral CP is limited.[127] The 10–20% false negative rate using EUS-FNA for resectable pancreatic cancer should not prohibit a patient from a potentially curative surgical procedure.[128] Sampling errors of EUS with EUS-FNA can occur because of the scant cellularity of specimens due to the small size of the lesions or the presence of CP. Other tumor-related factors may also decrease cellularity of samples, including extensive fibrosis (desmoplastic reaction) and necrosis, as well as the degree of differentiation (well-differentiated tumors require a larger number of needle passes then moderately or poorly differentiated tumors) [129, 130, 131, 132, 133, 134].

Power Doppler EUS in the Differentiation of Focal Chronic Pancreatitis and Pancreatic Adenocarcinoma

Power Doppler EUS also can provide useful information for the differential diagnosis of pancreatic masses. Saftoiu A et al. [127] included 42 consecutive patients with pancreatic tumor masses (27 men and 15 women) examined by EUS between January 2002 and August 2004. EUS procedures included power Doppler EUS as well as EUS-FNA in all patients. Final diagnosis of pancreatic cancer was confirmed in 29 patients on the basis of a combination of information provided by imaging tests, follow-up of at least 6 months, and laparotomy in 18 patients for diagnostic or palliative reasons. The results were in concordance with previous studies that showed a hypovascular pattern of pancreatic adenocarcinoma, as well as the formation of collaterals in advanced cases due to the invasion of the splenic or portal veins. Nonetheless, further studies of dynamic EUS with contrast agents are necessary to better characterize pancreatic masses. In their study [127], the ability of imaging methods (EUS with power Doppler imaging) was similar to that of EUS-FNA for the differential diagnosis of pancreatic cancer and pseudotumoral inflammatory masses. The addition of the information provided by the appearance of collaterals enhanced the diagnostic value of power Doppler ultrasonography, with better accuracy and a higher negative predictive value. Consequently, EUS with power Doppler imaging can provide information about the etiology of the tumor mass, even in the absence of tissue confirmation that may occur in patients with CP and pseudotumoral inflammatory masses. According to Saftoiu A et al. [127] the ability of power Doppler EUS to differentiate pancreatic masses has to be viewed as an adjunct to the other imaging techniques rather than a replacement of tissue confirmation. Currently, there is no imaging method that can reliably provide this capability in patients with pancreatic masses, especially in the setting of CP. Nevertheless, categorizing the risk of malignancy is very important for the clinical decision-making process and subsequent treatment (follow-up CT and EUS, repeated EUS-FNA, or surgery), especially in the cases with negative EUS-FNA findings, in which a diagnosis of pancreatic cancer cannot be excluded. Dynamic imaging is increasingly used for the differential diagnosis of pancreatic masses.[135] Pancreatic adenocarcinoma was described as usually hypovascular compared with the rest of the parenchyma, whereas inflammatory masses are isovascular or hypervascular. CE-EUS was also used for the differential diagnosis of pancreatic tumor masses for a better assessment of perfusion in the pancreatic tissue and inside the mass [136,137]. Pancreatic adenocarcinoma was shown to be relatively hypovascular compared with surrounding pancreatic tissue, whereas markedly hypervascular lesions were inflammatory masses. Although collaterals might also appear in CP because of segmentary portal hypertension, the relative frequency is inferior to the frequency of collateral appearance in patients with pancreatic cancer.[138] Consequently, combining the information provided by the absence of power Doppler signals and the presence of pancreatic collaterals yielded the best accuracy for the differential diagnosis between pseudotumoral CP and pancreatic adenocarcinoma.[127] Studies have shown comparable results with cytopathologic results (percutaneously or EUS-guided) with high sensitivity and specificity [137].

Chapter IV

Dorsal Extension of Resectable Pancreatic Cancer

The main role of staging pancreatic adenocarcinoma is to offer the most appropriate and stage-specific treatment strategy to the individual patient. The most critical issue is the accurate identification of patients that are eligible for complete resection, being those with no evidence of involvement of the superior mesenteric artery or celiac axis and of the superior mesenteric and portal venous (SMPV) confluence, in the absence of metastatic disease.

Important as well is the pre-operative assessment of the retroperitoneal margin (the soft tissue margin directly adjacent to the proximal 3-4 cm of the superior mesenteric artery) which is nearly always close and often positive. Its involvement, either by direct extension of the tumour or from retroperitoneal ExtraPancreatic Neural Invasion (EPNI) will in large part determine the likelihood of subsequent local recurrence in the pancreatic bed. Following intrapancreatic neural involvement cancer cells spread within the perineural space along the nerves, even as they branch, and infiltrate into surrouding connective tissue and likewise in the retroperitoneal space.[139, 140, 141, 142] EPNI clearly has to be distinguished from macroscopic invasion of adjacent neural tissue by the primary tumour, which overgrows neural tissues. It is not revealed by imaging studies like MRI and EUS, and in the clinicopathologic study of Nakao et al. EPNI independently and significantly correlated with a shortened postoperative survival.[140, 143] Levy and colleagues recently reported on the identification of microscopic EPNI by EUS-guided aspiration or biopsy examination in 2 patients with pancreatic adenocarcinoma. They stated that, although not a criterion considered in the current American Joint Committee on Cancer staging system, the preoperative finding of EPNI has the potential to alter patient management because it might influence the decision to resect, the extent of resection, and the administration of targeted adjuvant therapy to treat this hidden focus of disease [144].

Chapter V

Future Developments in the Diagnosis of Pancreatic Disease

In the future, age-related changes of the pancreatic parenchyma and its possible influence on the perfusion parameters need further investigation to optimise differentiation between different severities of CP and a "normal" higher age pancreatic parenchyma. In the elderly, pancreatic changes comparable to those occurring in patients with CP have been described. Further perfusion-based MRI studies are required to determine optimal models, and new software tools should be developed for clinical studies. Also, perfusion-based MRI has been used for the study of the pancreatic parenchyma [51] but has never been used in the differentiation between focal pancreatitis and a solid pancreatic tumor.

Ongoing developments in linear endoscopic ultrasound allowing better 3D view of the vessels near the pancreas might make early diagnosis and staging of pancreatic tumors more reliable. In a pilot study of 22 patients, the additional 3D reconstructions provided using linear EUS appeared to improve the evaluation of vessel-tumor relationships in pancreatic cancer, especially in case of CP. 3D imaging using linear EUS might have other applications but the acquisition system needs to be improved [145].

Other promising techniques are under development hopefully improving early differentiation between focal CP and pancreatic cancer. In vivo ^{1}H-MR spectra have been used showing significantly less lipid in focal CP than in pancreatic adenocarcinoma. The mean metabolite-to-lipid ratios were significantly different between pancreatic adenocarcinoma and focal CP; there was an overlap in the distribution of ratios between these 2 disease entities. This means that a misclassification should have existed. Further studies with larger sample sizes are needed to determine more specific criteria to predict each disease entity. Another possible limitation is the similarity of the assigned frequencies of the lipids and the lactate peaks on ^{1}H-MR spectra and the abundance of lipid molecules in the abdomen. For this reason, the application of MRS can be limited to the cases with a lesion large enough to contain the localization voxel. Further research to develop the new techniques of MRS that use the smaller localization voxel is required to eliminate this limitation [146].

Optical coherence tomography (OCT) using infrared light to produce two-dimensional images (1-2 mm in depth) analogous to ultrasound provides an exciting alternative means to identify ductal malignancy and comparative studies are eagerly awaited [147, 148, 149].

Conclusion

For the time being, differentiating between early CP and early pancreatic cancer still can be very difficult and sometimes impossible. Hopefully, many cases of unnecessary operation or delayed adequate treatment can be avoided by future developments allowing optimized diagnosis of pancreatic disease in an early stage.

References

[1] Sarner M. Pancreatitis: definitions and classification. In: Go V, editor. *The exocrine pancreas: biology, pathobiology, and diseases.* 2nd ed. New York: Raven; 1986; 459-464.

[2] Ritchie A. Pancreas. In: Ritchie A, editor. *Boyd's textbook of pathology.* 9th ed. Philadelphia: Lea and Febiger; 1990; 1202-1234.

[3] DiMagno E, Layer P, Clain J. Chronic pancreatitis. In: Go V, editor. *The pancreas: biology, pathology, and disease.* 2nd ed. New York: Raven; 1993; 665-706.

[4] DiMagno M, DiMagno E. Chronic Pancreatitis. *Curr. Opin. Gastroenterol.,* 2006; 22: 487-497.

[5] Sarles H. Proposal adopted unanimously by the participants of the Symposium, Marseilles 1963. *Bibl. Gastroenterol,* 1965; 7: 7-8.

[6] Sarner M, Cotton P. Classification of pancreatitis. *Gut,* 1984; 25: 756-759.

[7] Singer M, Gyr K, Sarles H. Revised classification of pancreatitis: report of the Second International Symposium on the Classification of Pancreatitis in Marseille, France, March 28-30, 1984. *Gastroenterology,* 1985; 89: 683-685.

[8] Sarles H, Adler G, Dani R, Frey C, Gullo L, Harada H, Martin E, Norohna M, Scuro L. The pancreatitis classification of Marseilles, Rome 1988. *Scand. J. Gastroenterol.,* 1989; 24: 641-642.

[9] Chari S, Singer M. The problem of classification and staging of chronic pancreatitis: proposal based on current knowledge and its natural history. *Scand. J. Gastroenterol.,* 1994; 29: 949-960.

[10] Ammann R. A clinically based classification system for alcoholic chronic pancreatitis: summary of an international workshop on chronic pancreatitis. *Pancreas,* 1997; 14: 215-221.
[11] Ramesh H. Proposal for a New Grading System for Chronic Pancreatitis. *J. Clin. Gastroenterol.*, 2002; 35: 67-70.
[12] Etemad B, Whitcomb D. Chronic pancreatitis: diagnosis, classification, and new genetic developments. *Gastroenterology*, 2001; 120: 682-707.
[13] Tandon R, Sato N, Carg P. For the consensus study group. Chronic pancreatitis: Asia-Pacific consensus report. *J. Gastroenterol Hepatol.*, 2002; 17: 508-518.
[14] Mallery J, Centeno B, Hahn P, Chang Y, Warshaw A, Brugge W. Pancreatic tissue sampling guided by EUS, CT/US, and surgery: a comparison of sensitivity and specificity. *Gastrointest Endosc.*, 2002; 56: 218-224.
[15] Kloppel G, Maillet B. A morphological analysis of 57 resection specimens and 9 autopsy pancreata. *Pancreas,* 1991; 6: 266-274.
[16] Lähr J. What are the useful biological and functional markers of early-stage chronic pancreatitis? *J. Gastroenterol.*, 2007; 42(Suppl 17): 66-71.
[17] Ito T. Can measurement of chemokines become useful biological and functional markers of early-stage chronic pancreatitis? *J. Gastroenterol.*, 2007; 42(Suppl 17): 72-77.
[18] Steer M, Waxman I, Freedman S. Chronic pancreatitis. *N. Engl. J. Med.*, 1995; 332:1482-1490.
[19] Catalano M, Lahoti S, Geenen J, Hogan W. Prospective evaluation of endoscopic ultrasonography, endoscopic retrograde pancreatography, and secretin test in the diagnosis of chronic pancreatitis. *Gastrointest Endosc.*, 1998; 48:11-17.
[20] Wiersema M, Hawes R, Lehman G, Kochman M, Sherman S, Kopecky K. Prospective evaluation of endoscopic ultrasonography and endoscopic retrograde cholangiopancreatography in patients with chronic abdominal pain of suspected pancreatic origin. *Endoscopy,* 1993; 25: 555-564.
[21] Feldman M, Friedman L, Sleisenger M. Pathophysiology, Diagnosis, Management. In: Saunders W, editor. *Sleisenger and Fordtran's Gastrointestinal and Liver Disease.* 7th ed. Philadelphia; 2002; 465-478.
[22] Niederau C, Grendell J. Diagnosis of chronic pancreatitis. *Gastroenterology,* 1985; 88: 1973-1995.

[23] Bastid C, Sahel J, Filho M, Sarles H. Diameter of the main pancreatic duct in chronic calcifying pancreatitis. Measurement by ultrasonography versus pancreatography. *Pancreas,* 1990; 5: 524-527.
[24] Raimondo M, Wallace M. Diagnosis of Early Chronic Pancreatitis by Endoscopic Ultrasound. Are We There Yet? *J. Pancreas*, 2004; 5: 1-7.
[25] Rajan E, Clain J, Levy M, Norton I, Wang K, Wiersema M, Vazquez-Sequeiros E, Nelson B, Jondal M, Kendall R, Harmsen S, Zinsmeister A. Age-related changes in the pancreas identified by EUS: a prospective evaluation. *Gastrointest Endosc.,* 2005; 61: 401-406.
[26] Ly J, Miller F. MR imaging of the pancreas: a practical approach. *Radiol. Clin. N. Am.,* 2002; 40: 1289-1306.
[27] Semelka R, Shoenut J, Kroeker M, Micflikier A. Chronic pancreatitis: MR imaging features before and after administration of gadopentetate dimeglumine. *JMRI,* 1993; 3: 79-82.
[28] Sica G, Braver J, Cooney M, Miller F, Chai J, Adams D. Comparison of endoscopic retrograde cholangiopancreatography with MR cholangiopancreatography in patients with pancreatitis. *Radiology*, 1999; 210: 605-610.
[29] Takehara Y, Ichijo K, Tooyama N, Kodaira N, Yamamoto H, Tatami M, Saito M, Watahiki H, Takahashi M. Breath-hold MR cholangiopancreatography with a long-echo-train fast spin-echo sequence and a surface coil in chronic pancreatitis. *Radiology,* 1994; 192: 73-78.
[30] Soto J, Barish M, Yucel E, Clarke P, Siegenberg D, Chuttani R, Ferrucci J. Pancreatic duct: MR cholangiopancreatography with a three-dimensional fast spin-echo technique. *Radiology,* 1995; 196: 459-464.
[31] Bret P, Reinhold C, Taourel P, Guibaud L, Atri M, Barkun A. Pancreas divisum: evaluation with MR cholangiopancreatography. *Radiology*, 1996; 199: 99-103.
[32] Miller F, Keppke A, Wadhwa A, Ly J, Dalal K, Kamler V. MRI of Pancreatitis and Its Complications: Part 2, Chronic Pancreatitis. *AJR,* 2004; 183: 1645-1652.
[33] Matos C, Metens T, Devière J, Niçaise N, Braude P, Van Yperen G, Cremer M, Struyven J. Pancreatic duct: morphologic and functional evaluation with dynamic MR pancreatography after secretin stimulation. *Radiology*, 1997; 203: 435-441.
[34] Cappeliez O, Delhaye M, Devière J, Le Moine O, Metens T, Niçaise N, Cremer M, Struyven J, Matos C. Chronic Pancreatitis: Evaluation of

Pancreatic Exocrine Function with MR Pancreatography after Secretin Stimulation. *Radiology,* 2000; 215: 358-364.
[35] Geenen J, Hogan W, Dodds W, Stewart E, Arndorfer R. Intraluminal pressure recording from the human sphincter of Oddi. *Gastroenterology,* 1980; 78: 317-324.
[36] Ochi K, Harada H, Mizushima T, Tanaka J, Matsumoto S. Intraductal secretin test is as useful as duodenal secretin test in assessing exocrine pancreatic function. *Dig. Dis. Sci.,* 1997; 42: 492-496.
[37] Wada K, Yamadera K, Yokoyama K, Goto M, Makino I. Application of pure pancreatic juice collection to the pancreatic exocrine function test. *Pancreas,* 1998; 16: 124-128.
[38] Gullo L, Costa P, Fontana G, Labo G. Investigation of exocrine pancreatic function by continuous infusion of caerulein and secretin in normal subjects and in chronic pancreatitis. *Digestion,* 1976; 14: 97-107.
[39] Gyr H, Agrawal N, Felsenfeld O, Font R. Comparative study of secretin and Lundh tests. *Am. J. Dig. Dis.,* 1975; 20: 506-512.
[40] Devière J, Gulbis B, Delhaye M, Quenon M, Cremer M. A study of the relationship between the canalar morphology and the exocrine function of the pancreas: a new method of linear estimation of the pancreatic function. *Acta Endosc.,* 1985; 15: 403-414.
[41] Hayakawa T, Kondo T, Shibata T, Noda A, Suzuki T, Nakano S. Relationship between pancreatic exocrine function and histological changes in chronic pancreatitis. *Am. J. Gastroenterol.,* 1992; 87: 1170-1174.
[42] Bozkurt T, Braun U, Leferink S, Gilly G, Lux G. Comparison of pancreatic morphology and exocrine functional impairment in patients with chronic pancreatitis. *Gut,* 1994; 35: 1132-1136.
[43] Malfertheiner P, Büchler M, Stanescu A, Ditschuneit H. Exocrine pancreatic function in correlation to ductal and parenchymal morphology in chronic pancreatitis. *Hepatogastroenterology,* 1986; 33: 110-114.
[44] Braganza J, Hunt L, Warwick F. Relationship between pancreatic exocrine function and ductal morphology in chronic pancreatitis. *Gastroenterology,* 1982; 82: 1341-1347.
[45] Otte M. Pankreasfunktionsdiagnostik. *Internist,* 1979; 20: 331-340.
[46] Matos C, Devière J, Cremer M, Niçaise N, Struyven J, Metens T. Acinar filling during secretin-stimulated MR pancreatography. *AJR,* 1998; 171: 165-169.
[47] Laugier R. Dynamic endoscopic manometry of the response to secretin in patients with chronic pancreatitis. *Endoscopy,* 1994; 26: 222-227.

[48] Karanjia N, Singh S, Widdison A, Lutrin F, Reber H. Pancreatic ductal and interstitial pressures in cats with chronic pancreatitis. *Dig. Dis. Sci.,* 1992; 37: 268-273.

[49] Reber H, Karanjia N, Alvarez C, Widdison A, Leung F, Ashley S, Lutrin F. Pancreatic blood flow in cats with chronic pancreatitis. *Gastroenterology,* 1992; 103: 652-659.

[50] Adler G, Schmid R. Chronic pancreatitis: still puzzling? *Gastroenterology,* 1997; 112: 1762-1765.

[51] Coenegrachts K, Van Steenbergen W, De Keyzer F, Vanbeckevoort D, Bielen D, Chen F, Dockx S, Maes F, Bosmans H. Dynamic contrast-enhanced MRI of the pancreas: initial results in healthy volunteers and patients with chronic pancreatitis. *JMRI,* 2004; 20: 990-997.

[52] Reber H, Karanjia N, Alvarez C, Widdison A, Leung F, Ashley S, Lutrin F. Pancreatic blood flow in cats with chronic pancreatitis. *Gastroenterology,* 1992; 103: 652-659.

[53] Patel A, Toyama M, Alvarez C, Nguyen T, Reber P, Ashley S, Reber H. Pancreatic interstitial pH in human and feline chronic pancreatitis. *Gastroenterology,* 1995; 109: 1639-1645.

[54] Lewis M, Lo S, Reber P, Patel A, Gloor B, Todd K, Toyama M, Sherman S, Ashley S, Reber H. Endoscopic measurement of pancreatic tissue perfusion in patients with chronic pancreatitis and control patients. *Gastrointest Endosc.,* 2000; 51: 195-199.

[55] Schilling M, Redaelli C, Reber P, Friess H, Signer C, Stoupis C, Buchler M. Microcirculation in chronic alcoholic pancreatitis: a laser Doppler flow study. *Pancreas,* 1999; 19: 21-25.

[56] Patel A, Reber P, Toyama M, Ashley S, Reber H. Effect of pancreaticojejunostomy on fibrosis, pancreatic blood flow, and interstitial pH in chronic pancreatitis. A feline model. *Ann Surg,* 1999; 230: 672-679.

[57] Verstraete K, Achten E, Dierick A. Dynamic contrast enhanced MRI of musculoskeletal neoplasms: different types and slopes of time-intensity curves (abstract). In: *Proceedings of the Society of Magnetic Resonance in Medicine;* Berkeley, California: Society of Magnetic Resonance in Medicine; 1992; 2609.

[58] Vaupel P, Kallinowski F, Okunieff P. Blood flow, oxygen and nutrient supply, and metabolic microenvironment of human tumors: a review. *Cancer Res.,* 1989; 49: 6449-6465.

[59] Kucharczyk J, Mintorovitch J, Asgari H, Moseley M. Diffusion/perfusion MR imaging of acute cerebral ischemia. *MRM,* 1991; 19: 311-315.

[60] Saeed M. Value of blood pool MR contrast agents in imaging of the heart and blood vessels. *Drugs Today*, 1999; 35: 879-892.

[61] Semelka R, Kroeker M, Shoenut J, Kroeker R, Yaffe C, Micflikier A. Pancreatic disease: prospective comparison of CT, ERCP, and 1.5-T MR imaging with dynamic gadolinium enhancement and fat suppression. *Radiology*, 1991; 181: 785-791.

[62] Winston C, Mitchell D, Outwater E, Ehrlich S. Pancreatic signal intensity on T1-weighted fat-saturation MR images: clinical correlation. *JMRI*, 1995; 5: 267-271.

[63] Zhang X-M, Shi H, Parker L, Dohke M, Holland G, Mitchell D. Suspected early or mild chronic pancreatitis: enhancement patterns on Gadolinium chelate dynamic MRI. *JMRI*, 2003; 17: 86-94.

[64] Sica G, Miller F, Rodriguez G, McTavish J, Banks P. Magnetic resonance imaging in patients with pancreatitis: evaluation of signal intensity and enhancement changes. *JMRI*, 2002; 15: 275-284.

[65] Prasad P, Wittmann J, Pereira S. Endoscopic Ultrasound of the Upper Gastrointestinal Tract and Mediastinum: Diagnosis and Therapy. *CVIR*, 2006; 29: 947-957.

[66] Sahai A, Zimmerman M, Aabakken L, Tarnasky P, Cunningham J, van Velse A, Hawes R, Hoffman B. Prospective assessment of the ability of endoscopic ultrasound to diagnose, exclude, or establish the severity of CP found by endoscopic retrograde cholangiopancreatography. *Gastrointest Endosc.*, 1998; 48:18-25.

[67] Sahai A. EUS and chronic pancreatitis. *Gastrointest Endosc.*, 2002; 56: S76-81.

[68] Vandervoort J, Soetikno R, Tham T, Wong R, Ferrari A, Montes H, Roston A, Slivka A, Lichtenstein D, Ruymann F, Van Dam J, Hughes M, Carr-Locke D. Risk factors for complications after performance of ERCP. *Gastrointest Endosc.*, 2002; 56: 652-656.

[69] Freeman M, DiSario J, Nelson D, Fennerty M, Lee J, Bjorkman D, Overby C, Aas J, Ryan M, Bochna G, Shaw M, Snady H, Erickson R, Moore J, Roel J. Risk factors for post-ERCP pancreatitis: a prospective, multicenter study. *Gastrointest Endosc.*, 2001; 54: 425-434.

[70] Wiersema M, Wiersema L. Endosonography of the pancreas: normal variation versus changes of early chronic pancreatitis. *Gastrointest Endosc. Clin. N. Am.*, 1995; 5: 487-496.

[71] Byrne M, Jowell P. Gastrointestinal imaging: endoscopic ultrasound. *Gastroenterology*, 2002; 122: 1631-1648.

[72] Lightdale C. Indications, contraindications, and complications of endoscopic ultrasonography. *Gastrointest Endosc,* 1996; 43: S15-19.

[73] Sahai A, Mishra G, Penman I, Williams D, Wallace M, Hadzijahic N, Pearson A, Vanvelse A, Hoffman B, Hawes R. EUS to detect evidence of pancreatic disease in patients with persistent or nonspecific dyspepsia. *Gastrointest Endosc.,* 2000; 52:153-159.

[74] Bhutani M. Endoscopic ultrasonography: changes of chronic pancreatitis in asymptomatic and symptomatic alcoholic patients. *J. Ultrasound Med.,* 1999; 18: 455-462.

[75] Kahl S, Glasbrenner B, Leodolter A, Pross M, Schulz H, Malfertheiner P. EUS in the diagnosis of early chronic pancreatitis: a prospective follow-up study. *Gastrointest Endosc.,* 2002; 55: 507-511.

[76] Yusoff I, Sahai A. A prospective, quantitative assessment of the effect of ethanol and other variables on the endosonographic appearance of the pancreas. *Clin. Gastroenterol. Hepatol,* 2004; 2: 405-409.

[77] Thuler F, da Costa P, de Paulo G, Nakao F, Ardengh J, Ferrari A. Endoscopic Ultrasonography and Alcoholic Patients: Can One Predict Early Pancreatic Tissue Abnormalities? *J. Pancreas*, 2005; 6: 568-574.

[78] Walsh T, Rode J, Theis B, Russell R. Minimal change chronic pancreatitis. *Gut,* 1992; 33: 1566-1571.

[79] Wallace M, Hawes R, Durkalski V, Chak A, Mallery S, Catalano M, Wiersema M, Bhutani M, Ciaccia D, Kochman M, Gress F, Van Velse A, Hoffman B. The reliability of EUS for the diagnosis of chronic pancreatitis: interobserver agreement among experienced endosonographers. *Gastrointest Endosc.,* 2001; 53: 294-299.

[80] Zimmermann M, Mishra G, Lewin D. Comparison of EUS findings with Histopathology in chronic pancreatitis [abstract]. *Gastrointest Endosc.,* 1997; 45: AB185.

[81] Hollerbach S, Klamann A, Topalidis T, Schmiegel W. Endoscopic ultrasonography (EUS) and fine-needle aspiration (FNA) cytology for diagnosis of chronic pancreatitis. *Endoscopy*, 2001; 33: 824-831.

[82] Hastier P, Buckley M, Francois E, Peten E, Dumas R, Caroli-Bosc F, Delmont J. A prospective study of pancreatic disease in patients with alcoholic cirrhosis: comparative diagnostic value of ERCP and EUS and long-term significance of isolated parenchymal abnormalities. *Gastrointest Endosc.,* 1999; 49: 705-709.

[83] Parada K, Peng R, Erickson R, Hawes R, Sahai A, Ziogas A, Chang K. A resource utilization projection study of EUS. *Gastrointest Endosc.,* 2002; 55: 328-334.
[84] Draganov P, Toskes P. Chronic pancreatitis. *Current opinion gastroenterol,* 2002; 18: 558-562.
[85] Jemal A, Murray T, Ward E, Samuels A, Tiwari R, Ghafoor A, Feuer E, Thun M. Cancer statistics, 2005. *CA Cancer J. Clin.,* 2005; 55: 10-30.
[86] Wiersema M. Accuracy of endoscopic ultrasound in diagnosing and staging pancreatic carcinoma. *Pancreatology,* 2001; 1: 625-632.
[87] Gress F, Gottlieb K, Sherman S, Lehman G. Endoscopic ultrasonography-guided fine-needle aspiration biopsy of suspected pancreatic cancer. *Ann Intern Med,* 2001; 134: 459-464.
[88] Moossa A, Gamagami R. Diagnosis and staging of pancreatic neoplasms. *Surg. Clin. North Am.,* 1995; 75: 871-890.
[89] DiMagno E, Reber H, Tempero M. AGA technical review on the epidemiology, diagnosis, and treatment of pancreatic ductal adenocarcinoma. American Gastroenterological Association. *Gastroenterology,* 1999; 117: 1464-1484.
[90] Trede M, Schwall G, Saeger H. Survival after pancreatoduodenectomy. 118 consecutive resections without an operative mortality. *Ann. Surg.,* 1990; 211: 447-458.
[91] Hawes R, Xiong Q, Waxman I, Chang K, Evans D, Abbruzzese J. A multispecialty approach to the diagnosis and management of pancreatic cancer. *Am. J. Gastroenterol.,* 2000; 95:17-31.
[92] Ahmad N, Lewis J, Ginsberg G, Haller D, Morris J, Williams N, Rosato E, Kochman M. Long term survival after pancreatic resection for pancreatic adenocarcinoma. *Am. J. Gastroenterol,* 2001; 96:2609-2615.
[93] Cameron J, Crist D, Sitzmann J, Hruban R, Boitnott J, Seidler A, Coleman J. Factors influencing survival after pancreaticoduodenectomy for pancreatic cancer. *Am. J. Surg.,* 1991; 161: 120-124.
[94] Sohn T, Yeo C, Cameron J, Koniaris L, Kaushal S, Abrams R, Sauter P, Coleman J, Hruban R, Lillemoe K. Resected adenocarcinoma of the pancreas-616 patients: results, outcomes, and prognostic indicators. *J. Gastrointest Surg.,* 2000; 4: 567-579.
[95] Richter A, Niedergethmann M, Sturm J, Lorenz D, Post S, Trede M. Long-term results of partial pancreaticoduodenectomy for ductal adenocarcinoma of the pancreatic head: 25-year experience. *World J. Surg.,* 2003; 27: 324-329.

[96] Pedrazzoli S, DiCarlo V, Dionigi R, Mosca F, Pederzoli P, Pasquali C, Kloppel G, Dhaene K, Michelassi F. Standard versus extended lymphadenectomy associated with pancreatoduodenectomy in the surgical treatment of adenocarcinoma of the head of the pancreas: a multicenter, prospective, randomized study. Lymphadenectomy Study Group. *Ann. Surg.*, 1998; 228: 508-517.

[97] Yeo C, Cameron J, Lillemoe K, Sohn T, Campbell K, Sauter P, Coleman J, Abrams R, Hruban R. Pancreaticoduodenectomy with or without distal gastrectomy and extended retroperitoneal lymphadenectomy for periampullary adenocarcinoma, part 2: randomized controlled trial evaluating survival, morbidity, and mortality. *Ann. Surg.*, 2002; 236: 355-366.

[98] DeWitt J, Devereaux B, Chriswell M, McGreevy K, Howard T, Imperiale T, Ciaccia D, Lane K, Maglinte D, Kopecky K, LeBlanc J, McHenry L, Madura J, Aisen A, Cramer H, Cummings O, Sherman S. Comparison of endoscopic ultrasonography and multidetector computed tomography for detecting and staging pancreatic cancer. *Ann. Intern. Med.*, 2004; 141: 753-763.

[99] Li D, Jiao L. Molecular Epidemiology of Pancreatic Cancer. *International Journal of Gastrointestinal Cancer*, 2003; 33: 3-13.

[100] Maitra A, Kern S, Hruban R. Molecular pathogenesis of pancreatic cancer. *Best Pract Res. Clin. Gastroenterol.*, 2006; 20: 211-226.

[101] Kloppel G. Pancreatic non-endocrine tumors. In: Kloppel G, Heitz PU, eds. *Pancreatic pathology*. Edinburgh: Churchill Livingstone; 1984; 87-88.

[102] Hosoki T. Dynamic CT of pancreatic tumors. *AJR,* 1983; 140: 959-965.

[103] Robbins S, Cotran R. The pancreas. In: Robbins SL, Cotran RS, eds. *Pathologic basis of disease*, 2nd ed. Philadelphia: Saunders; 1979: 1101-1102.

[104] Koito K, Namieno T, Nagakawa T, Morita K. Inflammatory Pancreatic Masses: Differentiation from Ductal Carcinomas with Contrast-Enhanced Sonography Using Carbon Dioxide Microbubbles. *AJR*, 1997; 169:1263-1267.

[105] Eloubeidi M, Chen V, Eltoum l, Jhala D, Chhieng DC, Jhala N, Vickers SM, Wilcox CM. Endoscopic ultrasound-guided fine-needle aspiration biopsy of patients with suspected pancreatic cancer: diagnostic accuracy and acute and 30-day complications. *Am. J. Gastroenterol.*, 2003; 98: 2663-2668.

[106] Fritscher-Ravens A, Brand L, Knofel W, Bobrowski C, Topalidis T, Thonke F, de Werth A, Soehendra N. Comparison of endoscopic ultrasound-guided fine needle aspiration for focal pancreatic lesions in patients with normal parenchyma and chronic pancreatitis. *Am. J. Gastroenterol.,* 2002; 97: 2768-2775.

[107] Farrell J. Diagnosing pancreatic malignancy in the setting of chronic pancreatitis: is there room for improvement? *Gastrointest Endosc.* 2005; 62: 737-741.

[108] Luetmar P, Stephens D, Ward E. Chronic pancreatitis: reassessment with current CT. *Radiology,* 1989; 171: 353–357.

[109] Müller M, Meyenberger C, Bertschinger P, Schaer R, Marincek B. Pancreatic tumors: evaluation with endoscopic US, CT, and MR imaging. *Radiology,* 1994; 190: 745–751.

[110] Johnson P, Outwater E. Pancreatic carcinoma versus chronic pancreatitis: dynamic MR imaging. *Radiology,* 1999; 212: 213-218.

[111] Lu D, Reber H, Krasny R, Kadell B, Sayre J. Local staging of pancreatic cancer: criteria for unresectability of major vessels as revealed by pancreatic-phase, thin section helical CT. *AJR,* 1997; 168: 1439-1443.

[112] Gabata T, Matsui O, Kadoya M, Yoshikawa J, Miyayama S, Takashima T, Nagakawa T, Kayahara M, Nonomura A. Small pancreatic adenocarcinomas: efficacy of MR imaging with fat suppression and gadolinium enhancement. *Radiology,* 1994; 193: 683-688.

[113] Van Hoe L, Gryspeerdt S, Marchal G, Baert A, Mertens L. Helical CT for the preoperative localization of islet cell tumors of the pancreas: value of arterial and parenchymal phase images. *AJR,* 1995; 165: 1437-1439.

[114] Elmas N. The role of diagnostic radiology in pancreatitis. *Eur. J. Radiol.,* 2001; 38:120-132.

[115] Friedman A. Pancreatic neoplasms and cysts. In: Friedman A, Dachman A, eds. *Radiology of the Liver, Biliary Tract, and Pancreas.* 1st ed. St. Louis: Mosby-Year Book; 1994; 807-934.

[116] Pamuklar E, Semelka R. MR imaging of the pancreas. *Magn. Reson. Imaging Clin. N. Am.*, 2005; 13: 313-330.

[117] Fayad L, Kowalski T, Mitchell D. MR cholangiopancreatography: evaluation of common pancreatic diseases. *Radiol. Clin. N. Am.*, 2003; 41: 97-114.

[118] Arslan A, Buanes T, Geitung J. Pancreatic carcinoma: MR, MR angiography and dynamic helical CT in the evaluation of vascular invasion. *Eur. J. Rad.,* 2001; 38: 151-159.

[119] Kim T, Murakami T, Takamura M, Hori M, Takahashi S, Nakamori S, Sakon M, Tanji Y, Wakasa K, Nakamura H. Pancreatic mass due to chronic pancreatitis: correlation of CT and MR imaging features with pathologic findings. *AJR*, 2001; 177: 367-371.

[120] Karawasa E, Goldberg H, Moss A, Federle M, London S. CT pancreatogram in carcinoma of the pancreas and chronic pancreatitis. *Radiology*, 1983; 148: 489-493.

[121] Ehnas N, Yoruhnaz I, Oran I, Oyar 0, Ozutemiz 0, Ozer H. A new criterion in differentiation of pancreatitis and pancreatic adenocarcinoma: artery-to-vein ratio using the superior mesenteric vessels. *Abdom. Imaging,* 1996; 21: 331-333.

[122] Ichikawa T, Sou H, Araki T, Arbab A, Yoshikawa T, Ishigame K, Haradome H, Hachiya J. Duct-penetrating sign at MRCP: usefulness for differentiating inflammatory pancreatic mass from pancreatic carcinomas. *Radiology*, 2001; 221: 107-116.

[123] Freeny P, Bilbao M, Katon R. Blind evaluation of endoscopic retrograde cholangiopancreatography (ERCP) in the diagnosis of pancreatic adenocarcinoma: the "double duct" and other signs. *Radiology*, 1976; 119: 271-274.

[124] Matos C, Bali M, Delhaye M, Devière J. Magnetic resonance imaging in the detection of pancreatitis and pancreatic neoplasms. *Best Pract. Res. Clin. Gastroenterol,* 2006; 20: 157-178.

[125] Remer E, Baker M. Imaging of chronic pancreatitis. *Radiol. Clin. North Am.,* 2002; 40:1229-1242.

[126] Lankish P. Function tests in the diagnosis of CP. *Int. J. Pancreatol.,* 1993; 14: 9-20.

[127] Saftoiu A, Popescu C, Cazacu S, Dumitrescu D, Georgescu C, Popescu M, Ciurea T, Gorunescu F. Power Doppler Endoscopic Ultrasonography for the Differential Diagnosis Between Pancreatic Cancer and Pseudotumoral Chronic Pancreatitis. *J. Ultrasound Med.,* 2006; 25: 363-372.

[128] Fickling W, Wallace M. Endoscopic ultrasound and upper gastrointestinal disorders. *J. Clin. Gastroenterol.,* 2003; 36: 103-110.

[129] Eloubeidi M, Jhala D, Chhieng D, Chen V, Eltoum I, Vickers S, Mel Wilcox C, Jhala N. Yield of endoscopic ultrasound-guided fine-needle aspiration biopsy in patients with suspected pancreatic carcinoma. *Cancer,* 2003; 99: 285-292.

[130] Vilmann P, Hancke S. A new biopsy handle instrument for endoscopic ultrasound guided biopsy. *Gastrointest Endosc.,* 1996; 43: 238-242.

[131] Erickson R. EUS-guided FNA. *Gastrointest Endosc.*, 2004; 60: 267-279.
[132] Itoi T, Itokawa F, Sofuni A, Nakamura K, Tsuchida A, Yamao K, Kawai T, Moriyasu F. Puncture of solid pancreatic tumors guided by endoscopic ultrasonography: A pilot study series comparing Trucut and 19-gauge and 22-gauge aspiration needles. *Endoscopy*, 2005; 37: 362-366.
[133] Wittmann J, Kocjan G, Sgouros S, Deheragoda M, Pereira S. Endoscopic ultrasound-guided tissue sampling by combined fine needle aspiration and trucut needle biopsy: A prospective study. *Cytopathology*, 2006; 17: 27-33.
[134] Ylagan L, Edmundowicz S, Kasal K, Walsh D, Lu D. Endoscopic Ultrasound Guided Fine-Needle Aspiration Cytology of Pancreatic Carcinoma. A 3-Year Experience and Review of the Literature. *Cancer*, 2002; 96: 362-369.
[135] Takhar A, Palaniappan P, Dhinga R, Lobo D. Recent developments in diagnosis of pancreatic cancer. *BMJ*, 2004; 329: 668-673.
[136] Bhutani M, Hoffman B, van Velse A, Hawes R. Contrast-enhanced endoscopic ultrasonography with galactose microparticles: SHU508A (Levovist). *Endoscopy*, 1997; 29: 635-639.
[137] Becker D, Strobel D, Bernatik T, Hahn E. Echo-enhanced and power Doppler EUS for the discrimination between focal pancreatitis and pancreatic carcinoma. *Gastrointest Endosc*, 2001; 53: 784-789.
[138] Eloubeidi M, Iseman D, Chen V, Vickers SM, Wilcox CM. Prevalence and significance of periduodenal venous collaterals in patients evaluated for pancreaticobiliary disorders by endosonography. *Endoscopy* 2003; 35:1015-1019.
[139] Ozaki H, Hiraoka T, Mizumoto R, Matsuno S, Matsumoto Y, Nakayama T, Tsunoda T, Suzuki T, Monden M, Saitoh Y, Yamauchi H, Ogata Y. The prognostic significance of lymph node metastasis and intrapancreatic perineural invasion in pancreatic cancer after curative resection. *Surg. Today*, 1999; 29: 16-22.
[140] Nagakawa T, Kayahara M, Ueno K, Ohta T, Konishi I, Ueda N, Miyazaki I. A clinicopathologic study on neural invasion in cancer of the pancreatic head. *Cancer*, 1992; 69: 930-935.
[141] Kayahara M, Nagakawa T, Futagami F, Kitagawa H, Ohta T, Miyazaki I. Lymphatic flow and neural plexus invasion associated with adenocarcinoma of the body and tail of the pancreas. *Cancer*, 1996; 78: 2485-2491.
[142] Takahashi T, Ishikura H, Kato H, Tanabe T, Yoshiki T. Intra-pancreatic, extra-tumoral perineural invasion. An indicator for the presence of

retroperitoneal neural plexus invasion by pancreatic adenocarcinoma. *Acta Pathol. Japonica*, 1992; 42: 99-103.

[143] Nakao A, Harada A, Nonami T, Kaneko T, Takagi H. Clinical significance of adenocarcinoma invasion of the extrapancreatic nerve plexus in pancreatic cancer. *Pancreas,* 1996; 12: 357-361.

[144] Levy M, Topazian M, Keeney G, Clain J, Gleeson F, Rajan E, Wang K, Wiersema M, Farnell M, Chari S. Preoperative Diagnosis of Extrapancreatic Neural Invasion in Pancreatic Cancer. *Clin. Gastroenterol. Hepatol,* 2006; 4: 1479-1482.

[145] Fritscher-Ravens A, Knoefel W, Krause C, Swain C, Brandt L, Patel K. Three-Dimensional Linear Endoscopic Ultrasound-Feasibility of a Novel Technique Applied for the Detection of Vessel Involvement of Pancreatic Masses. *Am. J. Gastroenterol.*, 2005; 100: 1296-1302.

[146] Cho S, Lee D, Lee K, Ji H, Lee K, Ros P, Suh C. Differentiation of Chronic Focal Pancreatitis From Pancreatic Carcinoma by In Vivo Proton Magnetic Resonance Spectroscopy. *JCAT,* 2005; 29: 163-169.

[147] Singh P, Chak A, Willis J, Rollins A, Sivak M. In vivo optical coherence tomography imaging of the pancreatic and biliary ductal system. *Gastrointest. Endosc., 2005;* 62: 970-974.

[148] Testoni P, Mangiavillano B, Albarello L, Arcidiacono P, Mariani A, Masci E, Doglioni C. Optical coherence tomography to detect epithelial lesions of the main pancreatic duct: an ex vivo study. *Am. J. Gastroenterol.*, 2005; 100: 2777-2783.

[149] Kwon R, Scheiman J. New Advances in Pancreatic Imaging. *Curr. Opin. Gastroenterol.*, 2006; 22: 512-519.

Index

A

abdomen, 60
abnormalities, 1, 3, 4, 15, 17, 69
accounting, 32
accuracy, 54, 71
acquisitions, 6, 13, 15
acute, 17, 20, 67, 71
Adams, 65
adenocarcinoma, 19, 26, 27, 31, 32, 47, 52, 54, 57, 59, 70, 71, 73, 74, 75
adenocarcinomas, 25, 32, 72
administration, 3, 4, 13, 58, 65
age, 2, 16, 17, 20, 59
agent, 7, 10, 12, 13, 14, 15, 27, 32, 33, 35, 36, 37, 38, 39, 40, 41, 42, 43, 45, 46, 48, 49, 52
agents, 14, 54, 68
aggressive behavior, 23
aid, 27, 52
alcohol, 18, 20
alcohol abuse, 18
alcohol use, 20
alcoholic cirrhosis, 21, 69
alcoholics, 20
alternative, 4, 60
anatomy, 17
angiography, 72
animal models, 5
animal studies, 6
animals, 13
aorta, 12
application, 20, 60
artery, 57, 73
Asia, 64
aspiration, 16, 26, 57, 69, 70, 71, 72, 73, 74
assessment, 4, 31, 55, 57, 68, 69
asymptomatic, 17, 20, 69
atrophy, 2, 3, 13, 26, 47
atypical, 49
autopsy, 64

B

Bali, 73
behavior, 23
benign, vii
bicarbonate, 5
bile, 2, 52
bile duct, 2, 52
biliary tract, 3, 4
biopsy, 1, 19, 57, 70, 71, 73, 74
blood, 13, 14, 25, 67, 68
blood flow, 13, 14, 25, 67
blood vessels, 68
blurring, 2
bolus, 12

bowel, 13, 19
breathing, 2, 12

C

calcification, 16, 26, 27, 52
caliber, 4, 52
California, 67
cancer, vii, 10, 23, 25, 26, 27, 31, 32, 36, 38, 42, 43, 52, 53, 54, 57, 59, 61, 70, 71, 72, 74, 75
cancer cells, 57
capillary, 14
carbon, 71
carcinoma, 70, 72, 73, 74
carcinomas, 73
cats, 67
cell, 19, 25, 72
cerebral ischemia, 67
certainty, 18
chemokines, 64
cholecystokinin, 13
chronic disease, 17
cirrhosis, 21, 69
classification, 1, 12, 20, 21, 63, 64
clinical oncology, 53
coherence, 60, 75
coil, 6, 65
collateral, 55
common bile duct, 52
communication, 19, 52
compliance, 5, 13
complications, 4, 68, 69, 71
composition, 14
computed tomography, 15, 71
concentration, 5, 35
concordance, 54
connective tissue, 57
consensus, 1, 64
contractions, 2
contrast agent, 7, 10, 12, 13, 14, 15, 27, 32, 33, 35, 36, 37, 38, 39, 40, 41, 42, 43, 45, 46, 48, 49, 52, 54, 68

control, 5, 15, 16, 20, 67
control group, 15
correlation, 5, 19, 66, 68, 73
cross-sectional, 20
cross-sectional study, 20
CT, 1, 4, 15, 16, 17, 19, 26, 27, 31, 32, 33, 39, 42, 43, 47, 48, 49, 54, 64, 68, 71, 72, 73
CT scan, 47
cyst, 44
cysts, 2, 16, 72
cytology, 16, 69

D

deaths, 23
decay, 2
decision-making process, 54
decompression, 14
demand, 21
density, 27
detection, 4, 5, 23, 52, 73
diet, 19
differential diagnosis, 26, 43, 53, 54
differentiation, vii, 10, 26, 27, 31, 52, 53, 59, 73
diffusion, 13, 39
dilation, 2, 19, 52
discrimination, 74
diseases, 15
displacement, 27
distribution, 1, 59
DNA, 25
DNA repair, 25
Doppler, 13, 54, 67, 73, 74
duodenostomy, 19
duodenum, 5
duration, 14
dyspepsia, 69

E

edema, 34, 35, 36
elasticity, 6, 13
elderly, 17, 59

Index

elderly population, 17
endocrine, 12, 71
endoscopic retrograde cholangiopancreatography, 64, 65, 68, 73
endoscopy, 17
enlargement, 3, 4, 26, 31, 52
enrollment, 20
enzyme, 19
epidemiology, 70
ethanol, 17, 31, 69
etiology, 54
evolution, 11
examinations, 20, 26, 27
exclusion, 36
exocrine, 4, 5, 12, 17, 63, 66

F

false negative, 53
fascia, 26
fat, 2, 3, 7, 10, 12, 14, 19, 26, 32, 35, 36, 37, 38, 40, 41, 45, 46, 52, 68, 72
FDG, 53
fibrosis, 3, 19, 25, 26, 27, 32, 47, 53, 67
fine needle aspiration, 16, 72, 74
flow, 4, 12, 13, 14, 25, 67, 74
fluid, 2, 3, 4, 6, 11, 26, 44
fluoroscopy, 17
FNA, 16, 20, 26, 53, 54, 69, 74
Fourier, 2, 6
France, 63

G

gadolinium, 3, 15, 47, 68, 72
gastrectomy, 71
gastrointestinal, 16, 17, 23, 73
gauge, 20, 74
gland, 2, 19, 47, 52
glucose, 12, 53
glucose tolerance, 12
glucose tolerance test, 12
gold, 1, 16, 19, 20, 21
gold standard, 1, 16, 19, 20, 21
grading, 1, 15
groups, 13, 18

H

hands, 23
health, 23
heart, 68
heterogeneous, 3
histological, 1, 18, 66
Holland, 68
human, 66, 67
humans, 5, 6
hypertension, 5, 55

I

identification, 57
images, 2, 3, 4, 6, 10, 14, 15, 17, 26, 32, 47, 60, 68, 72
imaging, vii, 1, 2, 3, 4, 6, 12, 13, 15, 16, 19, 23, 26, 31, 32, 35, 47, 54, 57, 59, 65, 67, 68, 72, 73, 75
imaging modalities, 1
imaging techniques, 1, 54
in situ, 31
inclusion, 12
indicators, 17, 70
infiltration, 48
inflammation, 1, 3, 32, 33
inflammatory, 25, 27, 32, 47, 52, 54, 73
infrared light, 60
ingestion, 18
injection, 4, 7, 10, 15, 17, 27, 32, 33, 35, 36, 37, 38, 39, 40, 41, 42, 43, 45, 46, 48, 49, 52
instruments, 16
intensity, 3, 6, 7, 8, 10, 11, 13, 14, 15, 31, 45, 67, 68
interstitial, 13, 14, 67
interval, 47
intervention, 4, 23
invasive, 5
Ireland, 12

ischemia, 67

L

laparotomy, 54
laser, 13, 67
leakage, 6
lesions, 1, 2, 16, 23, 53, 55, 72, 75
limitation, 60
limitations, 17
linear, 16, 59, 66
lipids, 59, 60
liver, 2
localization, 60, 72
London, 73
low fat diet, 19
lymph node, 74
lymphadenectomy, 71

M

Magnetic Resonance Imaging (MRI), 1, 2, 3, 4, 5, 6, 7, 10, 11, 13, 14, 15, 16, 26, 28, 29, 30, 31, 32, 34, 35, 36, 37, 38, 40, 41, 44, 45, 46, 47, 50, 51, 52, 57, 59, 65, 67, 68
malignancy, 31, 54, 60, 72
malignant, vii, 16
malignant tumors, 16
management, vii, 58, 70
measurement, 13, 64, 67
median, 20
mesenteric vessels, 73
metabolic, 53, 67
metabolic changes, 53
metabolite, 59
metastasis, 74
metastatic, 23, 57
metastatic disease, 57
microcirculatory, 13
microenvironment, 67
microparticles, 74
modalities, 1, 19
models, 5, 59
molecular biology, vii, 20

molecules, 60
morbidity, 23, 71
morphological, 15, 64
morphological abnormalities, 15
morphology, 17, 66
mortality, vii, 23, 70, 71
mortality rate, vii
motion, 2, 3
MRS, 60
musculoskeletal, 67
mutations, 25

N

NaCl, 12
natural, 20, 63
neck, 42, 43, 44
necrosis, 53
needle aspiration, 26, 69, 70, 71, 73
needles, 20, 74
neoplasms, 23, 67, 70, 72, 73
neoplastic, 25
nerves, 57, 75
Netherlands, 6
network, 14
neural tissue, 57
non-invasive, 6
normal, 2, 3, 4, 5, 6, 13, 14, 15, 16, 18, 19, 20, 21, 26, 32, 34, 35, 36, 37, 38, 52, 59, 66, 68, 72
nutrient, 67
nutrition, 19

O

obstruction, 4, 12, 25, 52
OCT, 60
oncological, 16
oncology, 53
optical, 75
oral, 12
oxygen, 67

P

pain, 19, 20, 64
palliative, 54
pancreas, 2, 3, 6, 12, 13, 16, 17, 18, 25, 31, 32, 47, 59, 63, 65, 66, 67, 68, 69, 70, 71, 72, 73, 74
pancreatectomy, 19
pancreatic, vii, 1, 2, 3, 4, 5, 6, 8, 10, 12, 13, 15, 16, 17, 19, 20, 21, 23, 25, 26, 27, 31, 32, 33, 34, 35, 36, 37, 38, 39, 40, 42, 43, 44, 45, 46, 47, 48, 49, 52, 53, 54, 57, 59, 61, 64, 65, 66, 67, 69, 70, 71, 72, 73, 74, 75
pancreatic acinar cell, 25
pancreatic cancer, vii, 10, 23, 25, 26, 27, 31, 36, 38, 42, 43, 52, 53, 54, 59, 61, 70, 71, 72, 74, 75
pancreatic duct, 2, 3, 4, 8, 16, 26, 27, 31, 32, 36, 38, 39, 40, 47, 52, 65, 67, 75
pancreatitis, vii, 1, 10, 12, 13, 14, 15, 17, 20, 21, 32, 41, 43, 44, 45, 52, 59, 63, 64, 65, 66, 67, 68, 69, 70, 72, 73, 74
parameter, 14
parenchyma, 3, 5, 6, 10, 13, 26, 27, 32, 34, 35, 36, 37, 38, 42, 45, 46, 47, 55, 59, 72
parenchymal, 1, 3, 17, 18, 26, 32, 66, 69, 72
parenchymal changes, 1
parenteral, 19
pathogenesis, 71
pathology, 42, 43, 63, 71
patient management, 58
performance, 68
perfusion, 6, 10, 13, 14, 55, 59, 67
permeability, 14
permit, 31
personal, 19
personal communication, 19
PET, 26, 53
pH, 67
Philadelphia, 63, 64, 71
pilot study, 59, 74
placebo, 19
plexus, 74, 75
poor, 17, 18, 23
population, 15, 18
portal vein, 12, 54
postoperative, 57
power, 54, 74
prediction, 19
pre-existing, 27
pressure, 6, 13, 66
prognosis, 23
protein, 3, 19, 35
protocol, 6, 13
proximal, 6, 34, 35, 36, 37, 38, 57
pseudocyst, 11

R

radiologists, 15
range, 3, 21
recognition, 3
reconstruction, 6
recurrence, 57
reduction, 14
relationship, 25, 66
reliability, 19, 69
repair, 25
research, 60
resection, 13, 19, 23, 26, 42, 53, 57, 58, 64, 70, 74
resolution, 3, 4, 13, 17
returns, 5
risk, 17, 18, 25, 54
risk factors, 17
ROI, 12
Rome, 1, 63

S

saline, 12
sample, 60
sampling, 5, 16, 64, 74
saturation, 68

Schmid, 67
secretin, 4, 5, 13, 18, 21, 64, 65, 66
secretion, 4
sedation, 17
sensitivity, 1, 2, 15, 18, 19, 26, 53, 55, 64
series, 6, 13, 23, 74
services, iv
severity, 20, 68
short-term, 20
sign, 28, 29, 30, 32, 50, 51, 52, 73
signals, 55
signs, 14, 15, 18, 32, 42, 43, 73
similarity, 60
SIR, 15
smoking, 17, 18
SNR, 2
software, 59
spatial, 3, 13
specificity, 1, 2, 15, 18, 20, 55, 64
spectrum, 31
speculation, 5
sphincter, 2, 4, 66
spin, 47, 65
stages, 5, 17
statistics, 70
stellate cells, 1
stenosis, 25
strictures, 4
structural changes, 18
suppression, 2, 3, 7, 10, 35, 36, 37, 38, 40, 41, 45, 46, 52, 68, 72
surgery, 12, 16, 23, 54, 64
surgical, 14, 19, 23, 26, 53, 71
surgical intervention, 23
surgical resection, 23, 26, 53
survival, 23, 57, 70, 71
survival rate, 23
susceptibility, 13
swelling, 25
symmetry, 2
symptoms, 19
systems, 1, 18

T

temporal, 13
therapy, 19, 58
three-dimensional, 65
threshold, 2, 10, 16, 18, 20
thresholds, 1
thrombosis, 12
TID, 13, 14
time, 4, 13, 14, 16, 19, 20, 23, 61, 67
tissue, 5, 6, 13, 14, 16, 17, 20, 26, 33, 48, 54, 57, 64, 67, 74
tissue perfusion, 6, 67
tolerance, 12
total parenteral nutrition, 19
training, 21
trial, 71
triggers, 1
triglycerides, 12
tumor, 23, 32, 53, 54, 57, 59
tumors, 16, 26, 32, 47, 53, 59, 67, 71, 72, 74
turnover, 25
two-dimensional, 60

U

ultrasonography, 54, 64, 65, 69, 70, 71, 74
ultrasound, 1, 15, 59, 60, 68, 70, 71, 72, 73, 74

V

values, 13, 16
variable, 26, 53
variables, 17, 69
variation, 68
vein, 12, 73
vessels, 14, 59, 68, 72, 73
visible, 15